Memory Bank for HIV Medications

Memory Bank for HIV Medications

GAIL M. WILKES RN, MS, OCN

Oncology Clinical Nurse Specialist
Boston City Hospital
Boston, Massachusetts

Jones and Bartlett Publishers
Boston   London

Editorial, Sales, and Customer Service Offices

Jones and Bartlett Publishers
One Exeter Plaza
Boston, MA 02116
1-617-859-3900
1-800-832-0034

Jones and Bartlett Publishers International
7 Melrose Terrace
London W6 7RL
England

Library of Congress Cataloging-in-Publication Data
Wilkes, Gail M.
    Memory bank for AIDS Medications / Gail M. Wilkes.
        p.   cm.
    Includes bibliographical references and index.
    ISBN 0-86720-685-3

    ISBN 13: 978-0-86720-685-2

    1. AIDS (Disease)--Chemotherapy--Handbooks, manuals, etc.
I.   Title
    [DNLM: 1. Acquired Immunodeficiency Syndrome--drug therapy-
-handbooks.   2. Anti-Infective Agents--handbooks. 3. Antineoplastic
Agents--handbooks.   WD 301 W682m 1994]
RC607.A26W527 1994
616.97'92061--dc20
DNLM/DLC
for Library of Congress   94-13546
                                                            CIP

Printed in the United States of America
98 97 96 95 94   10 9 8 7 6 5 4 3 2 1

Acquisitions Editor: Jan Wall
Production Editor: Joan M. Flaherty
Manufacturing Buyer: Dana L. Cerrito
Production Services and Typesetting: Total Concept
  Associates
Cover Design: Hannus Design Associates
Printing and Binding: InterCity Press
Cover Printing: Henry N. Sawyer Company

DISCLAIMER

Contents

Contents   *xi*

INTRODUCTION

This text is intended for the health care provider caring for persons with HIV (human immuno-deficiency virus) disease at any point along the health-illness continuum. As these individuals develop opportunistic infections and/ormalignancy, drug therapy becomes complex, and often the anti-infective agents may be confusing. Drugs well known in the past for treating obscure diseases, such as dapsone in the treatment of leprosy, now have regained prominence. Because quick, easy-to-retrieve information is necessary to sort through the many drugs the person with advanced HIV disease may be receiving, each drug is organized into concise sections: drug brand name, action, indications/uses, contraindications, dosage, administration, drug interactions, adverse affects, and nursing considerations/patient education. Key points are highlighted by bullets. Every attempt has been made to provide the most current, accurate information regarding the pharmacologic management of HIV-infected persons. This field is rapidly changing, however, and many clinical trials are ongoingto determine the most effective prophylactic and therapeutic regimens for many of the opportunistic infections and for HIV itself.

In order to provide a framework for the presentation of drugs used in the management of HIV disease, the first chapter reviews HIV disease.

Common opportunistic infections and malignancies are briefly reviewed in Chapter 2. Chapter 3 presents the drug profiles in alphabetical order. Drugs used in the treatment of HIV, opportunistic infections, malignancy, and symptom management are discussed. Because many persons, especially those with advanced HIV disease, receive multiple drugs, possible drug interactions are clearly indicated. Although chemotherapeutic agents used in the treatment of HIV-malignancies are included, these drugs should be administered by **specially trained nurses following established institutional guidelines for chemotherapy administration.** A bibliography completes the body of the text. The appendices include Occupational Safety and Health Administration (OSHA) guidelines for handling cytotoxic drugs, pharmacologic resources for indigent patients; average wholesaleprices at the time of publication for drugs used in HIV care; and quick references for calculation of absolute neutrophil count, crea-tinine clearance, and body surface area (BSA).

A comprehensive discussion of care of the person with HIV disease is beyond the scope of this pharmacologic text. Drugs contraindicated in pregnancy are indicated in the text. Although the Centers for Disease Control (CDC) has recommended that women with HIV infection should postpone childbearing until more is known about HIV transmission, some women may become pregnant. The incidence of HIV infection is increasing, and many of these women are in their reproductive years. Counseling is imperative, especially regarding the risks of transmission of HIV to the fetus, possible harm to the fetus if certain drug therapies become necessary for treatment of symptomatic infection in the mother, and possible impact of HIV illness on the mother and her child. A nonjudgmental approach should be employed. The likelihood that an HIV-infected mother will transmit the infection to her fetus (perinatal) is 25–35% (Ellerbrock and Rogers, 1990), but preliminary evidence suggests this risk is reduced by prophylaxis with zidovudine (AZT). Infection may also occur via the placenta or breast milk, and therefore, breast feeding of the infant is not advised. The mother's antibodies provide passive immunity for the newborn, so that the newborn possesses antibodies whether infected by the virus or not. Therefore, the HIV status of the newborn cannot generally be established before 15 months of age. Retrospective studies suggest that in asymptomatic mothers, pregnancy does not aggrevate HIV-infection in the mother. In contrast, Koonin et al (1989) found that in symptomatic HIV-infected mothers, there were increased maternal and fetal deaths.

In addition, all patients should be taught to avoid high-risk behaviors. Again, however, this book focuses on specific teaching related to each drug. General patient teaching information for persons with HIV infection can be found in other sources.

CHAPTER I

OVERVIEW OF HIV DISEASE

In the past decade, major pharmacologic advances have occurred to slow the progression from asymptomatic HIV infection to advanced acquired immune deficiency syndrome(AIDS). Unfortunately, to date, the antiretroviral agents prevent HIV replication only but do not eradicate the disease. The future is promising, as a variety of agents are currently being tested, including vaccines that may lead to disease prevention.

HIV disease begins with initial infection. HIV transmission occurs through intimate sexual contact; exposure to HIV-infected blood, blood products, or blood-containing body fluids; and maternal–fetal transmission. High-risk behaviors that place individuals at risk include homosexual sexual practices, unprotected heterosexual intercourse (oral, anal, or with multiple partners), and sharing equipment used for drug injection. In addition, children of HIV-infected mothers are at risk. Although intensive efforts to reduce high risk behavior have led to a decrease in the incidence of HIV infection in homosexual men, there is an increasing incidence in women.

The HIV virus selectively invades certain immune cells, principally the helper T- cell, which is integral to a competent immune system. The helper T-cells are called CD_4 cells because they have CD_4 receptors on the cell surface, which are targets for HIV binding. Other cells with CD_4 receptors are monocytes, macrophages, and certain brain cells, and thus these are targets for HIV as well. The HIV virion binds to the cell's CD_4 receptor, then fuses with the cell membrane and enters the host cell. HIV is a retrovirus with RNA in its nucleus. The virus RNA is uncoated, and, using the enzyme reverse transcriptase, synthesis of viral DNA occurs, which is then incorporated into the host cell's chromosomal DNA in the cell nucleus. The infected cell may remain quiescent or may be stimulated to divide, for example by infection. Once the cell is stimulated, viral DNA is activated, producing messenger RNA, which codes for the proteins necessary for viral replication. Synthesis of viral proteins occurs, and the viral protein coat and envelop as well as other elements are synthesized. The HIV virion is assembled in the host cell cytoplasm, and the virion "buds" off the host cell, releasing the HIV virion to infect other CD_4 cells. See Figure 1.1 for the HIV life cycle.

Antiretroviral agents such as zidovudine and didanosine are nucleoside analogues that inhibit reverse transcriptase, thus preventing HIV replication, viron release, and hence infection of other CD_4 receptor–bearing cells (T4 helper cell,

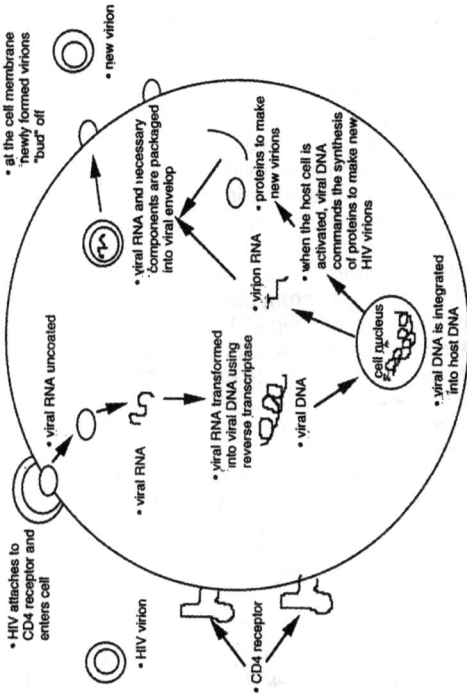

Figure 1.1   HIV Life Cycle

- HIV attaches to CD4 receptor and enters cell
- HIV virion
- CD4 receptor
- viral RNA uncoated
- viral RNA
- viral RNA transformed into viral DNA using reverse transcriptase
- viral DNA
- cell nucleus
- viral DNA is integrated into host DNA
- when the host cell is activated, viral DNA commands the synthesis of proteins to make new HIV virions
- virion RNA
- proteins to make new virions
- viral RNA and necessary components are packaged into viral envelop
- at the cell membrane newly formed virions "bud" off
- new virion

monocyte, macrophage). Persons with HIV disease show variability in disease progression, and studies have shown that persons with slower disease progression have stronger cytotoxic immune responses than those with rapid disease progression. The CD_4 cell count is a strong predictor of disease progression and mortality.

Clinically, once HIV transmission occurs, the person may experience a mononucleosis-like illness called acute retroviral infection, characterized by fever; adenopathy; sore throat; myalgia; and possibly rash, leukopenia, and hepatosplenism. This syndrome lasts one to two weeks; if laboratory testing is done, the individual would show high serum concentrations of HIV and a transient decrease in CD_4 cell count. Six to 12 weeks later, seroconversion occurs, and antibodies to the HIV p24 antigen are present. There is a marked decrease in HIV in the blood, and the CD_4 count returns to normal (Moss and Bacchetti, 1989).

Usually, the person experiences a period of asymptomatic infection, or may develop generalized lymphadenopathy. CD_4 counts gradually fall, from a normal value of around 1000/mm^3 to about 600–700/mm^3 during the first year of infection, then decreasing an average 50–80 CD_4 cells/mm^3 per year (Bartlett, 1992). As the CD_4 count falls below 500/mm^3, the person is at risk for the development of opportunistic infections and other conditions, such as *Herpes simplex* virus infection, oral candidiasis (thrush), vaginal candidiasis, hairy leukoplakia, shingles, idiopathic thrombocytopenia purpura, and pulmonary tuberculosis. Once the CD_4 count falls to $200/mm^3$, more severe opportunistic infections may occur, including *Pneumocystis carinii* pneumonia, *Candida* esophagitis, toxoplasmosis encephalitis, cryptococcal meningitis, cryptosporidiosis, chronic mucocutaneous *Herpes simplex* virus, and others. As the CD_4 count falls to less than $50-100/mm^3$, *Mycobacterium avium* complex (MAC) and disseminated *cytomegalovirus* (CMV) may occur, as well as lymphoma. This progression of HIV disease in relation to falling CD_4 counts is depicted in Figure 1.2. In addition, clinical syndromes such as HIV wasting and dementia may occur. Table 1.1 shows the Centers for Disease Control (CDC) AIDS case definitions.

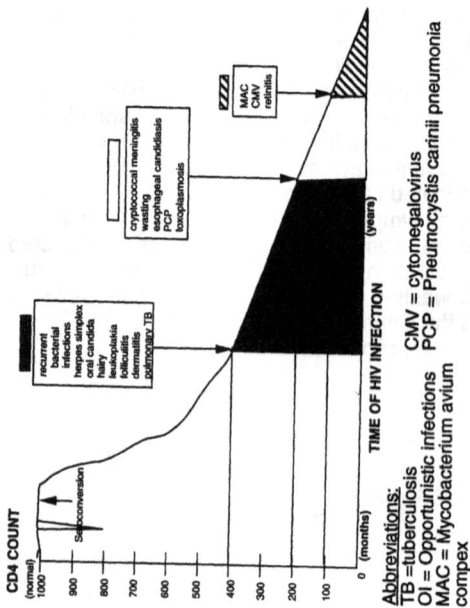

CD4 COUNT
(normal)

Seroconversion

recurrent
bacterial
infections
herpes simplex
oral candida
hairy
leukoplakia
folliculitis
dermatitis
pulmonary TB

cryptococcal meningitis
wasting
esophageal candidiasis
PCP
toxoplasmosis

MAC
CMV
retinitis

TIME OF HIV INFECTION

(months)   (years)

Abbreviations:
TB = tuberculosis   CMV = cytomegalovirus
OI = Opportunistic infections PCP = Pneumocystis carinii pneumonia
MAC = Mycobacterium avium
compex

Figure 1.2   Development of Oppurtunistic
Infections as CD4 Count Falls

Memory Bank for HIV Medications

Table 1.1   1993 revised classification system for HIV infection and expanded AIDS surveillance case definition for adolescents and adults*

	Clinical categories		
	(A)	(B)	(C)
CD4 + T=cell categories	Asymptomatic acute (primary) HIV or PGL**	Symptomatic not (A) or (C) conditions**	AIDS-indicator conditions**
(1) ≥/µL	A1	B1	
(2) 200–499/µL	A2	B2	
(3) <200/µL AIDS-indicator T-cell count	A3	B3	C3

*The shaded cells illustrate the expanded AIDS surveillance case definition. Persons with AIDS-indicator conditions (Category C) as well as those with CD4+ T-lymphocyte counts 200/µL (Categories A3 or B3) will be reportable as AIDS cases in the United States and Territories, effective January 1, 1993.

**PGL=persistent generalized lymphadenopathy. Clinical Category A includes acute (primary) HIV infection (29,30).

Category A

Category A consists of one or more of the following conditions in an adolescent or adult (≥ 13 years) with documented HIV infection. Conditions listed in Categories B and C must not have occurred.

- Asymptomatic HIV infection
- Persistent generalized lymphadenopathy
- Acute (primary) HIV infection with accompanying illness or history of acute HIV infection (29,30)

Category B
Category B consists of symptomatic conditions in an HIV-infected adolescent or adult that are not included among conditions listed in clinical Category C and that meet at least one of the following criteria: (a) the conditions are attributed to HIV infection or are indicative of a defect in cell-mediated immunity; or (b) the conditions are considered by physicians to have a clinical course or to require management that is complicated by HIV infection. **Examples** of conditions in clinical Category B include, **but are not limited to:**

- Bacillary angiomatosis
- Candidiasis, oropharyngeal (thrush)
- Candidiasis, vulvovaginal; persistent, frequent, or poorly responsive to therapy
- Cervical dysplasia (moderate or severe)/ cervical carcinoma in situ
- Constitutional symptoms, such as fever (38.5℃) or diarrhea lasting > 1 month
- Hairy leukoplakia, oral
- Herpes zoster (shingles), involving at least two distinct episodes or more than one dermatome

- Idiopathic thrombocytopenic purpura
- Listeriosis
- Pelvic inflammatory disease, particularly if complicated by tubo-ovarian abscess
- Peripheral neuropathy

Category C
- Candidiasis of bronchi, trachea, or lungs
- Candidiasis, esophageal
- Cervical cancer, invasive
- Coccidioidomycosis, disseminated or extrapulmonary
- Cryptococcosis, extrapulmonary
- Cryptosporidiosis, chronic intestinal (>1 month's duration)
- Cytomegalovirus disease (other than liver, spleen, or nodes)
- Cytomegalovirus retinitis (with loss of vision)
- Encephalopathy, HIV-related
- Herpes simplex: chronic ulcer(s) (> 1 month's duration); or bronchitis, pneumonitis, or esophagitis
- Histoplasmosis, disseminated or extrapulmonary
- Isosporiasis, chronic intestinal (> 1 month's duration)
- Kaposi's sarcoma
- Lymphoma, Burkitt's (or equivalent term)
- Lymphoma, immunoblastic (or equivalent term)
- Lymphoma, primary, of brain
- Mycobacterium avium complex or *M. kansasii,* disseminated or extrapulmonary

- *Mycobacterium tuberculosis,* any site (pulmonary or extrapulmonary)
- *Pneumocystis carinii* pneumonia
- Pneumonia, recurrent
- Progressive multifocal leukoencephalopathy
- *Salmonella* septicemia, recurrent
- Toxoplasmosis of brain
- Wasting, syndrome due to HIV

Reproduced from U.S. Department of Health and Human Services, Public Health Service, Centers for Disease Control (1992) "1993 Revised Classification System for HIV Infection and Expanded Surveillance Case Definition for AIDS Among Adolescents and Adults" *Morbidity and Mortality Weekly Report* 41 (RR–17): 1–16

In the past it was common practice in the United States to begin antiretroviral therapy early, in the hope of delaying the occurrence of opportunistic infections. However, it was unclear which agent was best, or whether overall survival was affected. Results of AIDS clinical trial group (ACTG) protocols 016 and 019 showed that zidovudine (AZT) delayed progression of HIV disease to AIDS and the development of opportunistic infections in individuals with early HIV infection and CD_4 counts <500/mm^3 (Volberding et al, 1990). As a result of this study, zidovudine therapy was recommended for symptomatic and asymptomatic HIV-infected persons whose CD_4 counts were < 500/mm^3 (Consensus Group, 1990). However, no survival advantage has been shown, and investigators of the Concorde I study, a collaborative British–French effort, recommended antiretroviral therapy be deferred until symptoms arise (Aboulker and Swart, 1993). There are concerns about the Concorde I study methodology, and current studies are ongoing to confirm optimal time to initiate treatment and potential survival benefits of early therapy. It is anticipated that guidelines for antiretroviral therapy will change as current clinical trials are completed. At this time, antiretroviral therapy with zidovudine may be initiated in patients with CD_4 counts < 500/mm^3, or providers may wish to delay therapy until patients are symptomatic or CD_4 counts are < 200/mm^3. Zidovudine is the preferred antiretroviral agent; didanosine is considered when patients have toxicity from zidovudine or develop resistance (disease progression). Combination therapy with zidovudine and zalcitabine (ddC) or didanosine (ddI) is controversial, and is considered for patients with advanced disease or for those who have received zidovudine for an extended period of time and may be developing resistance (Volberding, 1992).

As HIV disease progresses, CD_4 counts continue to fall to 0–50/mm^3. Most deaths from HIV disease occur during this period of advanced

HIV infection. Patients may experience a wasting syndrome, thought to be due to HIV-stimulated tumor necrosis factor (cachexin), and other symptoms such as pain, anorexia, and fatigue may occur. Helping patients to optimize their quality of life becomes the major challenge for clinicians during the most advanced stage of HIV infection.

CHAPTER 2

OPPORTUNISTIC INFECTIONS AND MALIGNANCY

Opportunistic infections that complicate HIV infection are often caused by organisms that are commonly found in our everyday environment and have low pathogenicity to healthy people. Because of the HIV-infected individual's immune deficiency, these organisms may create potentially serious, life-threatening infections. Causative organisms are bacterial, viral, fungal, and parasitic/protozoal.

BACTERIAL INFECTIONS
Major *bacterial* infections include tuberculosis and *Mycobacterium avium* complex.

Tuberculosis (TB) is caused by the acid-fast *Mycobacterium tuberculosis*, and can result in *infection* or *active disease*. Infection occurs following airborne transmission of the bacteria into the body, and an intact immune system ensures that the number of TB bacteria is small, causing no harm to the individual. During this time, the bacteria are dormant, and although the individual tests positive for PPD (Purified Protein Derivative skin testing), the individual has no symptoms and is not infectious (is unable to transmit the bacteria to others). However, during times of diminished immune function, the TB bacilli may become reactivated and may cause active disease. In contrast, active disease occurs when an individual's immune system is unable to eliminate the bacteria, and a largre number of the TB bacilli cause signs and symptoms of TB disease: fatigue, malaise, weight loss, fever, night sweats, and lymphadenopathy. These individuals not only show a positive PPD skin test and symptoms of TB, but also may have an abnormal chest X-ray and may be contagious. Both groups usually require medications to eliminate the TB bacilli.

Since 1985, there has been an increased incidence of active tuberculosis (TB) and increasing rates of resistance to isoniazid (INH) and rifampin, the most effective agents for treatment of TB. One of the factors responsible for the emergence of multidrug resistance to TB is incomplete treatment, so that the TB organism is no longer sensitive to conventional treatment and behaves in a much more aggressive manner. In communities with high rates of HIV, up to 40% of patients with active TB are HIV-infected, and those infected by resistant strains have a high mortality.

Clinical presentation of TB in HIV-infected persons may be atypical and may involve extrapulmonary sites. The cell-mediated immune system is responsible for eliminating the TB bacilli. In HIV-infected individuals, this system becomes inadequate, as evidenced by decreasing CD_4 counts. Often patients with CD_4 counts of approximately 200/mm^3 are *anergic* (e.g., unable to mount an immune response, so there is an absence of normal skin reaction to a PPD challenge or to other proteins the body has encountered in the past). Thus, controls (for example *Candida albicans,* mumps) must be planted with the PPD (purified protein derivative). If there is no skin reaction to the PPD, then that individual could either: (a) have no previous TB infection or (b) have TB infection but be so immunologically compromised that the body cannot mount a response (false negative test). Therefore, placing intradermal controls, such as mumps or *Candida,* on an individual's opposite arm will help determine whether the individual is truly anergic or is PPD negative.

Patients at risk for developing TB should receive INH prophylaxis (INH 300 mg/day plus pyridoxine) for 12 months. However, chest X-ray must be obtained first. Also, if the patient is coughing, active disease must first be ruled out by three negative culture and sensitivities. Those at risk are HIV-positive individuals with a positive PPD (> 5 mm induration) and those who are anergic and are IV drug users, homeless, natives of an endemic country, or otherwise at risk. All anergic patients should receive a screening chest X-ray. Most providers treat TB in AIDS patients with a 9–12 month or longer regimen including isoniazid (INH), rifampin, ethambutol, and pyrazinamide. Patients infected by resistant strains are treated with at least two active drugs (e.g., ciprofloxacin or ofloxacin and ethambutol or pyrazinamide) and should be followed by a pulmonary or infectious disease specialist. When culture and sensitivities show resistance to a drug(s), **two drugs** must be added to the failing regime. Patients who are directly observed in self-administration of the medications may often be more compliant. After two months of therapy, most anti-TB regimens can be modified to three times a week dosing, thereby improving compliance.

Mycobacterium avium complex (MAC) includes infections caused by *Mycobacterium avium* and the related *Mycobacterium intracellulare* (MAI), common bacteria found in soil and water, which are harmless to immunocompetent individuals. However, in HIV-infected persons with CD_4 counts $< 100/mm^3$, disseminated infection can occur, involving any organ. Often the lungs, liver, bone marrow, and lymph nodes are affected, and at least 50% of HIV-infected persons will become infected by MAC. Symptoms include constitutional symptoms (fever, fatigue, night sweats, weight loss) and anemia; when the GI tract is involved, abdominal pain and diarrhea can occur. Clinical trials are underway to determine the most effective prophylactic regimen. Rifabutin (300 mg q day) is indicated for prophylaxis of MAC, and other agents with possible effectiveness include azithromycin and clarithromycin. No optimal regimen is available to treat existing infection, so treatment is not usually given unless the patient is symptomatic. Drugs being studied in treatment of MAC are clarithromycin or azithromycin plus ethambutol plus: rifampin or rifabutin, or clofazimine or ciprofloxacin.

Most important of the other bacterial infections are recurrent bacterial pneumonias, which confer a diagnosis of AIDS in an HIV-infected individual. Pneumonia most often is caused by *Pneumonococci, Staphlococci, and Streptococci.* Thus, the Centers for Disease Control (CDC) recommend pneumoncoccal vaccinations (e.g., pneumovax) for individuals who are HIV-infected (CDC, 1989), as well as influenza vaccine, since these individuals are at increased risk (CDC, 1992). Other common bacterial infections experienced by HIV-infected persons include those caused by *Klebsiella, Enterobacter, Shigella, and Salmonella,* Listeriosis. The sexually transmitted diseases caused by *Chlamydia trachomatis* and *Neisseria gonorrhaeae* are also common.

VIRAL INFECTIONS
Opportunistic viral infections include those caused by *Herpes simplex* virus (HSV), *Cytomegalovirus* (CMV), and *Varicella zoster* virus.

Herpes simplex viral (HSV) infections are often persistent, become severe, and involve multiple mucocutaneous sites such as those in the mouth, esophagus, and rectum. Thus, HSV infections are aggressively treated to prevent systemic progression and to enhance quality of life.

Acyclovir is used topically, orally, or parenterally. Following initial treatment, patients may receive secondary prophylaxis to prevent recurrence. This is a controversial area, since drug resistance may develop and benefit must be weighed carefully against risks. Foscarnet can be used to treat resistant HSV strains.

CMV is a ubiquitous herpes virus that threatens the vision and life of HIV-infected patients. Infection can involve any organ, but most severe are infections of the retina (CMV retinitis) and colon (CMV colitis). Thus, all patients with CD_4 counts $< 100/mm^3$ must have an ophthalmologic exam every six months to screen for CMV retinitis. Ganciclovir is used initially and for posttreatment suppression of CMV retinitis that must be continued lifelong. G-CSF (Granulocyte-Colony Stimulating Factor, filgrastim) or GM-CSF (Granulocyte-Macrophage Colony Stimulating Factor, sargramostim) is often necessary to prevent neutropenia. For those patients whose CMV retinitis progresses on treatment, Dietrich et al (1993) have demonstrated efficacy of combination therapy using foscarnet and ganciclovir. A prospective, randomized clinical trial is now being conducted.

Shingles, caused by *Varicella zoster* virus, may occur early or late in the spectrum of HIV infection, and frequently is disseminated. Severe infections involving more than one dermatome, disseminated, or involving the trigeminal nerve are treated with intravenous acyclovir at higher doses than those for *Herpes simplex* infection for 7–14 days, or with foscarnet for 14–26 days in patients resistant to acyclovir. Treatment must begin within 72 hours. Less severe infection is treated with oral acyclovir for 7–10 days.

Other viral infections are those caused by the Human papilloma virus (HPV), which causes genital warts and is implicated in the increased risk of cervical cancer in HIV-infected women, and in homosexual men, anal squamous carcinoma; *molluscum contagiosum* virus; and Epstein-Barr virus, which causes hairy leukoplakia. Women with lifestyle behaviors that put them at risk should receive annual routine screening for cervical cancer (for example Papanicolaou test), gonorrhea, and *Chlamydia*. Finally, hepatitis is common in many HIV-infected individuals, who are at great risk to become chronic hepatitis B carriers. Thus, hepatitis B vaccine is often recommended (Hadler, 1988).

FUNGAL INFECTIONS
The most common fungal infections are candidiasis, cryptococcosis, and histoplasmosis.

Oral candidiasis (thrush) in an otherwise healthy individual may be the first sign of HIV infection. *Candidia* species are common, and infection of mucocutaneous membranes can include those of the oral cavity, esophagus, intestines, or bladder, or the fungus can disseminate systemically. Esophageal candidiasis is an AIDS-defining diagnosis. Ketoconazole, an oral antifungal azole drug, is often ineffective in HIV-infected patients because the drug requires an acid pH, and often these individuals are achlorhydric (having little or no gastric acid), thus preventing drug absorption. Fluconazole is the antifungal treatment of choice for mucosal infections. Systemic, invasive, or resistant infections are treated with intravenous Amphotericin B.

Cryptococcus neoformans occurs commonly in the environment (soil, pigeon feces), and 10–12% of patients with advanced HIV infection will develop cryptococcal meningitis, an AIDS-defining diagnosis. The patient often presents with gradual onset of fever and headache, occurring in the late afternoon. Other signs and symptoms include nausea, vomiting, photophobia, altered mental status, and seizures. Fluconazole is used to treat mild to moderately severe infections (400 mg orally every day for 6–10 weeks) followed by lifetime suppressive treatment (100–200 mg daily). Severe or resistant infections require Amphotericin B induction for 2–4 weeks, followed by lifetime fluconazole suppressive therapy. Interestingly, patients may receive fluconazole to prevent recurrent Candidal infections, and this may also provide prophylaxis for cryptococcal meningitis as well. Prophylactic regimens include fluconazole

50–100 mg daily, itraconazole 100 mg daily, or ketoconazole 200 mg daily.

Infection caused by *Histoplasma capsulatum* confers a diagnosis of AIDS. It is more common in HIV-infected individuals living or traveling to the central United States, Latin America, or the Caribbean, where the fungus is endemic. The patient may have constitutional signs of malaise, fever, chills, weight loss, fatigue, as well as abdominal pain, lymphadenopathy, and hepatosplenomegaly. Intravenous Amphotericin B or oral itraconazole, followed by lifetime suppressive therapy are the most commonly used agents.

PARASITIC AND PROTOZOAN INFECTIONS
Finally, parasitic and protozoan infections represent the final group of opportunistic infections.

Pneumocystis carinii pneumonia (PCP) is the most common and most important opportunistic infection in this class, affecting an estimated 80% of patients with advanced HIV disease who do not receive prophylaxis. Prophylaxis is recommended for patients with CD_4 counts $\leq$ 200 cells/mm^3, and trimethoprim-sulfamethoxazole (TMP-SMX, Bactrim®) is currently the drug of choice, one tablet given every day or one double strength (DS) tablet three times weekly. In addition, this drug offers prophylaxis against infections caused by bacteria and toxoplasmosis. Since HIV-infected patients have more toxicity from TMP-SMX and may be unable to tolerate the drug, Dapsone 100 mg orally twice a week may be offered as an alternative prophylactic regimen. A comparative trial comparing TMP-SMX, dapsone, and aerosolized pentamidine is now underway. Aerosolized pentamidine is less favored by many because of its inability to provide drug to the lung apices consistently, so that relapse may occur here; the inability to provide prophylaxis against systemic or extrapulmonary infections caused by *Pneumocystis carinii*; and the inability to prophylaxe against other opportunistic infections caused by bacteria or toxoplasmosis. In addition, it is more expensive. Treatment of active PCP usually involves TMP-SMX, atovaquone (Mepron®), or oral dapsone with or without trimethoprim for 21-day therapy. Parenteral pentamidine, with or without prednisone, is used for more severe infection. Alternative therapy includes clindamycin and primaquine for 21 days.

Toxoplama gondii is the causative agent in toxoplasmosis, and this organism is often carried by domestic cats. Patients with advanced HIV disease may present with encephalitis or a mass lesion in the central nervous system (CNS). Signs and symptoms include fever, headache, change in mental status, sensory loss, paralysis, and seizures. HIV-related CNS lymphoma may also present this way and must be excluded in the differential diagnosis. This is often accomplished

through empiric combination therapy for toxoplasmosis with pyrimethamine and sulfadiazine for
6 weeks. In general, most (> 90%) of patients will
have a clinical response within two weeks, which
confirms the diagnosis. Otherwise, a brain biopsy
must be performed. Alternative therapies include
pyrimethamine and clindamycin; or azithromycin
and pyrimethamine; or atovaquone. Continued
lifelong suppressive therapy is necessary. As
previously mentioned, prophylactic PCP therapy
with TMP-SMX or dapsone also provides
prophylaxis for toxoplasmosis.

OPPORTUNISTIC MALIGNANCY
As patients live longer with deliberate prophylaxis
against many of the opportunistic infections,
opportunistic malignancies may develop, or they
may be the presenting symptoms to confer an
AIDS diagnosis. The most common malignancies
are Kaposi's sarcoma and non-Hodgkin's
lymphoma (NHL).

Kaposi's sarcoma (KS) was often considered
synonymous with an AIDS diagnosis, since when
AIDS was first described, KS and *Pneumocystis
carinii* pneumonia (PCP) were the major AIDS-
defining diagnoses. In the past, the classic form of
this disease was well described in men from the
Mediterreanean area. In this population, KS is a
slow-growing, fairly benign disease. In contrast,
the "epidemic" KS seen in HIV-infected individuals
is more variable and aggressive (Cooley, 1993).

KS was long considered a malignancy, but today some experts say it is an inflammatory response to angiogenic stimulation, mediated by cytokines and the tat gene (Vogel, 1988). Although the incidence of KS has declined (Rutherford et al, 1989), KS is still most common in HIV-infected homosexual or bisexual men and is uncommon in women. Palpable, violaceous (red, blue, or purple) cutaneous or mucocutaneous lesions may appear on the face, palate, legs, feet, or rectum. Diagnosis is made by punch biopsy. The clinical disease spectrum ranges from asymptomatic, with isolated cutaneous lesions, to a highly aggressive, rapidly fatal disease. More aggressive or more advanced tumors often affect the viscera, causing symptoms depending on the involved site, such as bleeding (e.g., gastrointestinal lesions), or dyspnea (e.g., pleural effusions and pulmonary lesions). Patients with the best prognosis have lesions confined to skin or to lymph nodes, or have minimal oral disease; have CD_4 counts > $200/mm^3$; and have no previous opportunistic infections or thrush, no "B" symptoms of weight loss, fevers, or night sweats; and a Karnofsky performance status $\geq$ 70% (E.g., is able to care for self, but cannot do normal activity/work.) (Krown et al, 1989).

Local therapy for painful or large cutaneous lesions is palliative, and includes radiotherapy, and intralesional chemotherapy. Interferon-alpha is effective in 30–50% of patients with high CD_4

counts, and cutaneous lesions (Groopman et al, 1989). Systemic therapy for progressive or advanced disease employs low-dose or nonmyelosuppressive chemotherapy, since often these patients have HIV-related or anti-retroviral-related neutropenia or thrombocytopenia.

Commonly used regimens are:

- Weekly IV vincristine (1.5–2.0 mg/week)
- Weekly IV vinblastine (0.05–0.1 mg/kg or 3 mg/m^2 per week, if absolute neutrophil count (ANC) > 1000/mm^3)
- IV vincristine (1.5–2.0 mg/week alternating with IV vinblastine (0.05–0.1 mg/kg or 3 mg/m^2) every other week
- Vincristine 2 mg IV and Bleomycin 10u/m^2 IV, every 14 days
- Biweekly (every 14 days) ABV for advanced, symptomatic disease:

    —Doxorubicin 10–20 mg/m^2 IV

    —Bleomycin 10 u/m^2 IV

    —Vincristine 1.0–2.0 mg IV

ABV chemotherapy appears to be most effective, with response rates of 45–88% and median survival of 9 months (Gill et al, 1991). Response rates may be increased when combined with zidovudine or with zidovudine and GM-CSF; studies are ongoing to confirm this, as well as to determine the efficacy of ABV in combination with didanosine (ddl) or dideoxycytidine (ddC) by the AIDS clinical trial group (ACTG).

Therapy is palliative, and although quality of life appears to be markedly improved, survival is not prolonged.

HIV lymphoma is most often a high-grade B-cell lymphoma, and is a non–Hodgkin's type (NHL), although Hodgkin's disease does occur. The etiology of AIDS-related NHL is unclear, but it may be caused by chronic viral antigenic and mitogenic stimulation of the immune system, leading to overproduction of B-cell lymphocytes (Yarchoan et al, 1986). Most patients present with extensive disease; up to 85% of patients have extranodal disease, involving the bone marrow, CNS, GI tract, liver, or even soft tissues such as the breast or pancreas. Poor prognostic features are extranodal disease, previous AIDS diagnosis, CD_4 count < 100 cells/mm^3, and a poor performance status. Patients with total CD_4 count above 100/mm^3 survive longer (4.5 months versus 24 months) as reported by Kaplan (1989). Aggressive therapy with full or modified doses is required, and necessitates the addition of granulocyte-colony Stimulating factor (G-CSF, filgrastim) or granulocyte-macrophage colony-stimulating factor (GM-CSF, sargramostim) to prevent life-threatening febrile neutropenia. Granulocyte-macrophage-colony stimulating factor (GM-CSF, sargramostim) will stimulate the release of HIV from infected macrophages and must be given concomitantly with an antiretroviral agent. Complications of treatment include opportunistic infections and severe bone marrow depression (Cooley, 1993). CNS sterilization with intrathecal chemotherapy is performed to prevent CNS relapse. Levine (1989) reported a 46% complete response rate using low-dose m-BACOD chemotherapy, CNS prophylaxis, and zidovudine maintenance. Currently, an AIDS clinical trial group (ACTG) is comparing low-dose m-BACOD to standard dose m-BACOD (doxorubicin 45mg/m^2, cyclophosphamide 600mg/m^2) with GM-CSF 20 μg/kg SC days 3–13 of each cycle (Cooley, 1993). This should clarify whether there is a survival advantage to using higher chemotherapy doses.

Chemotherapy regimens include modified m-BACOD (methotrexate-bleomycin, Adriamycin®, cyclophosphamide, Oncovin® and dexamethasone); and modified CHOP, given less frequently, if at all (cyclophosphamide, H = doxorubicin, Oncovin®, prednisone).

- **m-BACOD**, given every 21 days for 4–6 cycles (low-dose)
    - Day 1: Bleomycin 4 units/m^2 IV
      Doxorubicin (Adriamycin®) 25 mg/m^2 IV
      Cyclophosphamide 300 mg/m^2 IV
      Vincristine (Oncovin®) 1.4mg/m^2 IV (max 2.0 mg)
      dexamethasone 3mg/m^2 PO days 1–5

Day 15:   methotrexate 200 mg/m^2 IV with leukovorin rescue 25 mg PO q 6 hours X 6 beginning 24 hours after methotrexate

CNS sterilization with cytosine arabinoside 50 mg intrathecally X 4 in first month; if CNS has lymphoma cells, radiotherapy given as well

- **Modified CHOP**, every 21 days for 4–6 cycles

  Day 1:   Cyclophosphamide 400–500 mg/m^2 IV

  Doxorubicin (Adriamycin®) 25–30 mg/m^2 IV

  Vincristine (Oncovin®) 1.4 mg/m^2 IV

  Prednisone 100 mg/m^2 PO d1–5

- **CHOP**, every 21 days for 4–6 cycles

  Day 1:   Cyclophosphamide 750 mg/m^2 IV

  Doxorubicin (Adriamycin®) 50 mg/m^2 IV

  Vincristine (Oncovin®) 1.4 mg/m^2 IV

  Prednisone 100 mg/m^2 PO d1–5

GM-CSF or G-CSF day starting 24 hours after chemotherapy X 10 days

CHAPTER 3

DRUG PROFILES

Acetaminophen

BRAND NAME:
- Tylenol; also, many other products, including pharmacy brand name products and combination preparations with other drugs

ACTION:
- Nonnarcotic analgesic; inhibits prostaglandin synthesis centrally; reduces fever through effect on hypothalamus

INDICATIONS:
- Mild pain, fever

CONTRAINDICATIONS:
- Known hypersensitivity
- Use cautiously if at all in patients with severe hepatic or renal dysfunction

DOSAGE:
- 325–650 mg q 4–6 hours prn pain
- max dose: 4 gm/24 hours

ADMINISTRATION:
- Oral (tablets or elixir)
- Rectal suppositories

DRUG INTERACTIONS:
- Alcohol: increased hepatotoxicity
- Barbiturates, carbamazepine, rifampin, phenytoin: may increase acetaminophen serum levels when drug used chronically; monitor for hepatotoxicity
- Diflunisal: increases acetaminophen serum level; avoid concurrent use

ADVERSE EFFECTS:
- Uncommon with therapeutic dosing
- Pruritis, maculopapular rash
- Sensitivity

SPECIAL NURSING CONSIDERATIONS:
- Elixir contains alcohol
- May mask fever curve or excessive fever
- Monitor baseline and periodic liver function tests, especially if patient is taking large doses of acetaminophen or if patient has preexisting liver dysfunction
- Some preparations contain sulfites; patients with sulfite allergies should read drug label carefully
- Overdose may be fatal

PATIENT EDUCATION:
- Report fever over 101º F, or persistent or recurrent fever

- Report all medications taken, include over-the-counter medications that may also contain acetaminophen
- Avoid excessive alcohol ingestion
- Avoid overdosage

Acyclovir

BRAND NAME:
- Zovirax

ACTION:
- Antiviral agent; prevents replication of *Herpes Simplex virus* (HSV), and *Varicella zoster* virus

INDICATIONS:
- Initial and recurrent mucosal and cutaneous *Herpes simplex* infections (HSV-1, HSV-2), and acute *Herpes zoster*

CONTRAINDICATIONS:
- Known hypersensitivity
- Use with caution in patients receiving nephrotoxic drugs or who are pregnant, or nursing
- Use IV drug with caution in patients who developed neurotoxicity after intrathecal methotrexate

DOSAGE:
- Mucocutaneous HSV infection: 5 mg/kg IV q 8 hours X 7 days or 200 mg PO 5 X/day X 10 days; consider posttreatment suppression with 200–400 mg PO bid
- Herpes zoster: within 72 hours: severe, > one dermatome, or disseminated:
  10–12 mg/kg IV q 8 hours X 7–14 days
  not severe: 800 mg po 5 X/day X 7 days
- Varicella (chickenpox): 10–12 mg/kg IV q 8 hours X 7 days or until clinical improvement
- Dose reduce if renal dysfunction exists or occurs

ADMINISTRATION:
- Oral, Intravenous, or as an ointment
- Administer IV over AT LEAST ONE HOUR AND ENSURE ADEQUATE HYDRATION and urine elimination for 2 hours after dose

DRUG INTERACTIONS:
- Amphotericin B: potentiates antiretroviral activity of acyclovir
- Interferon: synergism
- Probenecid:↑acyclovir serum levels
- Zidovudine: may potentiate antiretroviral activity of zidovudine

ADVERSE EFFECTS:
* *Uncommon:*
  —Fever, headache
  —Confusion, paresthesias, visual abnormalities
  —Rash, pruritis

—Transient ↑ in BUN, serum creatinine
—Diarrhea, increased liver function tests, nausea

SPECIAL NURSING CONSIDERATIONS:
• Monitor BUN, serum creatinine baseline and during IV acyclovir therapy
• Patients with large HSV mucocutaneous ulcers may become resistant, and require second-line foscarnet therapy
• Minimal injury to normal cells so few adverse effects

PATIENT EDUCATION:
• Self-administration of oral drug
• Chronic suppressive therapy after initial therapy for mucocutaneous HSV in HIV-infected individuals is often necessary

Alprazolam

BRAND NAME:
• Xanax

ACTION:
• Anxiolytic agent; binds to receptors in CNS to bring about anxiety reduction and muscle relaxation

INDICATIONS:
• Anxiety, panic attacks

CONTRAINDICATIONS:
- Known hypersensitivity to drug
- Depressive neuroses, psychotic reactions, acute closed-angle
  Glaucoma
- Pregnancy, nursing mothers
- Use cautiously in patients with liver or renal dysfunction, chronic pulmonary disease, or sleep apnea

DOSAGE:
- *Adult:* anxiety: 0.25–0.5 mg PO tid (can titrate up to maximum 4 mg/day); to be used for short-term effect only
- Discontinue drug by reducing dose by 0.25–0.5 mg q 3–7 days when used for extended periods

ADMINISTRATION:
- Oral; may take with food to reduce stomach upset

DRUG INTERACTIONS:
- Alcohol, anticonvulsants, opiates, phenothiazines: additive CNS depression; use together cautiously and monitor closely
- Oral contraceptives, isoniazid, ketoconazole, cimetidine: decreased plasma clearance of alprazolam with increased sedation; monitor patient closely
- Tricyclic antidepressants: increased alprazolam serum level; use together cautiously

- Digoxin: may decrease excretion of digoxin; monitor serum digoxin level and modify dose as needed

ADVERSE EFFECTS:
- CNS depressant effects (drowsiness, fatigue, lethargy, weakness, headache, confusion)
- *Less common:*
  - —Nausea, vomiting, constipation
  - —Hypotension
  - —Urticaria, rash

SPECIAL NURSING CONSIDERATIONS:
- Drug has anticonvulsant properties
- Drug can cause psychologic and physical dependency
- Discontinue drug if manic episodes or hyperactivity occur after drug initiated
- Withdrawal symptoms can occur with rapid drug discontinuance when drug is taken for extended periods or in high doses
- Discontinue drug and refer for psychiatric assessment if patient expresses suicidal thoughts
- Drug has high "street drug value" as it potentiates effects of methadone, heroin and other opiates

PATIENT EDUCATION:
- Use drug only when needed for a short time, NOT to manage everyday stress

Drug Profiles

- Drug may impair ability to drive a car or ability to work with heavy machinery, so do not perform these activities when taking the drug
- Stop drug if hyperactivity or manic feelings occur when drug initiated
- Avoid taking alcohol when receiving this drug

Amikacin Sulfate

BRAND NAME:
- Amikin

ACTION:
- Aminoglycoside antibiotic, active against many gram-negative and some gram-positive bacteria

INDICATIONS:
- Bacterial sepsis
- Serious infections of respiratory tract, bones and joints, CNS, skin, soft tissues, intra-abdominal infections

CONTRAINDICATIONS:
- Known hypersensitivity to drug or to other aminoglycosides
- Pregnancy, nursing mothers

DOSAGE:
- 15 mg/kg/day in divided doses q 8–12 hours IV or IM to attain peak serum concentration of 15–30 µg/mL, and trough serum concentration of 5–10 µg/mL
- Dose must be reduced in renal dysfunction

ADMINISTRATION:
- IV: dilute in 100–200 mL IV fluid, infuse over 30–60 minutes
- IM: into large muscle mass such as gluteus maximus

DRUG INTERACTIONS:
- Aminoglycosides, amphotericin B, bacitracin, cisplatin, furosemide, vancomycin: increases risk of ototoxicity; avoid concurrent use
- Succinyl choline, tubocurarine: potentiates neuromuscular blockade; use cautiously
- Extended-spectrum penicillins: synergism; must be administered separately

ADVERSE EFFECTS:
- Ototoxicity with dizziness, nystagmus, vertigo, tinnitus
- Nephrotoxicity
- Headache, tremor, lethargy
- Rash, urticaria, pruritis, fever
- Nausea, vomiting, anorexia (rare)

SPECIAL NURSING CONSIDERATIONS:
- May cause superinfection by nonsusceptible organisms such as *Candida*

- Assess BUN, creatinine baseline, and monitor daily during therapy
- Assess serum levels (peak 30–90 minutes after dose and trough just prior to next dose) during therapy
- Dose reduction necessary for renal dysfunction
- Ensure adequate hydration
- Use in treatment of resistant TB should be in consultation with physician expert in the management of resistant TB

PATIENT EDUCATION:
- Report changes in hearing ability (tinnitus, decreased hearing)
- Increase oral fluids
- Report vaginal itching or discharge (females), or thrush (white spots on oral mucosa)

Amoxicillin / Clavulanate Potassium

BRAND NAME:
- Augmentin

ACTION:
- Antibiotic agent with beta-lactamase inhibitor, preventing development of drug resistance

INDICATIONS:
- Infections caused by susceptible organisms in the lower respiratory tract, ear (otitis media), sinus, skin/skin structures, urinary tract

CONTRAINDICATIONS:
- Hypersensitivity
- History of allergic reactions to penicillins
- Use cautiously in patients with multiple allergies or allergy to cephalosporins

DOSAGE:
- *Adult and children > 40 kg:* 250 mg q 8 hours; for more serious infections, 500 mg q 8 hours
- *Children ≤ 40 kg:* 20 mg/kg/day–40 mg/kg/day in divided doses every 8 hours
- MODIFY DOSE IF RENAL DYSFUNCTION

ADMINISTRATION:
- Oral without regard to meals
- Augmentin 250 tablet contains 125 mg clavulanic acid, and should be used for adults and children weighing ≥ 40 kg. Chewable 250 mg tablet contains 62.5 mg clavulanic acid and should be used for children weighing < 40 kg

DRUG INTERACTIONS:
- Allopurinol: may increase incidence of rash; use together cautiously
- Disulfiram: AVOID CONCURRENT USE

ADVERSE EFFECTS:
- Diarrhea/loose stools, nausea, vomiting
- Skin rash, urticaria
- Vaginitis
- Rarely, pseudomembranous colitis

SPECIAL NURSING CONSIDERATIONS:
- Discontinue drug if rash or serum sickness (rash, urticaria plus arthralgias, myalgias, fever) develop
- Immunocompromised patients may develop positive Coombs' test (direct antiglobin)

PATIENT EDUCATION:
- Stop drug and report rash, arthralgias, fever, persistent or severe diarrhea

Amphotericin B

BRAND NAME:
- Fungizone

ACTION:
- Antifungal agent; damages fungal membran

INDICATIONS:
- Systemic fungal infections caused by *Asper lus, Candida, Cryptococcus, Histoplasma capsulatum*, and fungal meningitis

CONTRAINDICATIONS:
- Known hypersensitivity to drug

- Use with caution in renal dysfunction, pregnancy

DOSAGE:
- Initial (test dose): 0.25 mg/kg IV (or first dose 1 mg IV) over 2–6 hours
- Gradually increase daily dose to 0.5–1 mg/kg/day (or 1.5 mg/kg when given on alternate days)
- If dose interrupted for > 1 week, reinstitute at 0.25 mg/kg/day and titrate up
- Intrathecal: 25 µg (0.1 mL diluted with 10–20 mL cerebrospinal fluid) 2–3 X per week

ADMINISTRATION:
- Use PRESERVATIVE-FREE diluent in reconstituting drug
- Intravenous: administer slowly over 2–6 hours; if in-line filter used, must be ≥ 1µm or drug will be filtered out; protect from light during infusion
- Intrathecal

DRUG INTERACTIONS:
- Norfloxacin: possible enhanced antifungal action
- Aminoglycosides, cisplatin, cyclosporine, pentamidine, vancomycin: additive nephrotoxic effects; avoid concurrent administration
- Corticosteroids: enhanced hypokalemic effects
- Digitoxin: enhanced toxicity related to amphotericin-induced hypokalemia

- Flucytosine: synergism with increased drug effect
- Miconazole: antagonism; do not use together
- Nitrogen mustard: increases toxicity (renal, bronchospasm, hypotension); avoid concurrent administration
- Granulocyte transfusions: acute pulmonary dysfunction may occur if given concurrently or close together. Time administration far apart and monitor pulmonary function

ADVERSE EFFECTS:
- Headache, hypotension, malaise, myalgias, tachypnea
- Nausea, vomiting, cramping
- Fever, chills 1–3 hours after infusion begins
- Nephrotoxicity, hypokalemia
- Reversible normocytic, normochromic anemia
- Rare hypertension, cardiac arrest, pulmonary edema, bronchospasm
- After IT administration, headache, visual changes, neck stiffness

SPECIAL NURSING CONSIDERATIONS:
- Tolerance to drug occurs over time, with reduction in fever, chills
- Assess temperature, vital signs baseline and frequently during infusion
- Discuss premedication with physician to prevent rigors: ibuprofen or acetaminophen; diphenhydramine, IV meperidine; and/or hydrocortisone

- Monitor BUN, serum creatinine, and potassium baseline and at least every other day during dosage escalation, then weekly
- Ensure adequate hydration: monitor intake, output, and total body fluid balance closely
- Replace potassium as ordered
- Monitor CBC baseline and during treatment
- Change IV site daily or q 48 hours; apply heat to increase comfort during infusion. Infuse drug SLOWLY

PATIENT EDUCATION:
- Report fever, chills, dyspnea, other side effects immediately
- Increase oral fluid intake
- Report phlebitis immediately

Ampicillin

BRAND NAMES:
- Omnipen, Polycillin, Principen

ACTION:
- Penicillin antibiotic that inhibits bacterial cell wall synthesis

INDICATIONS:
- Infections of upper and lower respiratory tract, genitourinary tract, skin by sensitive organisms

CONTRAINDICATIONS:
- Known hypersensitivity to penicillins
- Use with caution in patients hypersensitive to cephalosporin antibiotics

DOSAGE:
- *Adult:*
  - —Oral: 250–500 mg q 6 hours
  - —IM/IV: 2–12 gm q d in 4–6 divided doses
- Dose modification if renal dysfunction

ADMINISTRATION:
- Oral: administer 1 hour before meals or 2 hours after meals
- IM/IV

DRUG INTERACTIONS:
- Aminoglycoside antibiotics: synergism
- Rifampin: possible antagonism at high doses of penicillin
- Probenecid: increases serum levels of ampicillin
- Oral contraceptives: may decrease efficacy; women should use alternative contraceptive measures

ADVERSE EFFECTS:
- *Common:*
  - —Rash, urticaria
  - —Overgrowth of nonsusceptible organisms (e.g., *Candida*)
- *Less common:*
  - —Vomiting, glossitis

—Blood dyscrasias
—Stevens-Johnson syndrome

SPECIAL NURSING CONSIDERATIONS:
- Rarely, pseudomembranous colitis caused by *Clostridium difficile* occurs. If diarrhea is persistent or severe, drug should be stopped. Often, this is sufficient to resolve diarrhea
- Fungal superinfection may occur, such as vaginal moniliasis in women

PATIENT EDUCATION:
- Report rash to physician or nurse
- Take drug 1 hour before meals or 2 hours after meals
- Assess for signs/symptoms of (super)infection
- Report persistent or severe diarrhea

Aspirin (Acetylsalicylic acid)

BRAND NAMES:
- Aspergum, ASA, Bayer Aspirin, Ecotrin

ACTION:
- Antipyretic, antiinflammatory, nonnarcotic analgesic; exerts effect through inhibition of prostaglandin synthesis

INDICATIONS:
- Fever; mild to moderate pain, especially joint or bone pain

CONTRAINDICATIONS:
- Known hypersensitivity
- Receiving myelosuppressive chemotherapy
- GI ulcer, GI bleeding, bleeding tendency
- Use cautionly in patients with asthma, rhinitis, or nasal polyps (can cause bronchospasm)
- Use cautiously in patients with liver dysfunction, thrombocytopenia

DOSAGE:
- 325–650 mg PO or PR q 4 hours, prn
- MAX 3.9 gm/day

ADMINISTRATION:
- Oral; rectal suppository
- Give oral dose with large glass of water, milk, or food to reduce gastric irritation
- Do not crush enteric coated aspirin

DRUG INTERACTIONS:
- Ammonium chloride, ascorbic acid, or methionine (urine acidifiers): decrease ASA excretion so increase risk of ASA toxicity
- Antacids, urinary alkalizers: may increase ASA excretion so may decrease the ASA effect.
- Alcohol increases the risk of GI ulceration, bleeding
- Beta-adrenergic blockers (e.g., propranolol): possible decrease in antihypertensive effect
- Coumarin: increase prothrombin time; DO NOT USE CONCURRENTLY

- Corticosteroids: increase in aspirin excretion with decrease in aspirin effect
- Methotrexate: increase in MTX serum levels with increased toxicity. Do not use concurrently
- NSAIDs: decrease in NSAID serum concentration; may have increased incidence of GI side effects. Do not use together
- Probenecid, sulfinpyrazone: aspirin (doses > 3 gm/day) antagonizes uricosuric drug effect
- Spirolactone: aspirin may inhibit diuretic effect
- Sulfonylyreas, exogenous insulin: aspirin may have hypoglycemic effect and may potentiate these drug actions; monitor for hypoglycemia.
- Valproic acid: aspirin displaces drug and decreases its excretion, resulting in increased serum levels and possible valproic acid toxicity

ADVERSE EFFECTS:
- Nausea, heartburn, epigastric discomfort, acute reversible liver toxicity
- Bleeding, especially if large doses administered
- Mild salicylism: dizziness, tinnitus, decreased hearing, nausea, vomiting, diarrhea, mental confusion, headache, sweating, hyperventiliation

SPECIAL NURSING CONSIDERATIONS:
- Oral solution can be made from Alka-Seltzer
- Salicylism occurs with serum salicylate levels 150–300 μg/mL. Serum level with usual dosing is 100 μg/mL

PATIENT EDUCATION:
- Take with food or milk
- Signs/symptoms of salicylism, and to reduce or discontinue aspirin if these occur
- Discontinue drug if bleeding or black stools occur and notify physician or nurse

Atovaquone

BRAND NAME:
- Mepron

ACTION:
- Antiprotozoal agent

INDICATIONS:
- Oral treatment of mild to moderate *Pneumocystis carinii* pneumonia in patients unable to tolerate trimethoprim-sulfamethoxazole (TMP-SMX)

CONTRAINDICATIONS:
- Known hypersensitivity to the drug
- Pregnant women or breast-feeding mothers unless benefit outweighs risk

DOSAGE:
- 750 mg tid X 21 days

ADMINISTRATION:
- Available in 250 mg tablets
- Administer with food

DRUG INTERACTIONS:
- Drug is highly protein-bound and will compete with other highly plasma protein-bound drugs

ADVERSE EFFECTS:
- Rash (23%)
- Nausea (21%)
- Diarrhea (19%)
- Fever (14%)
- Insomnia (10%)
- Asthenia (8%)
- Liver dysfunction (rare)
- Headache (16%)

SPECIAL NURSING CONSIDERATIONS:
- Drug has a 30% failure rate
- Useful in the treatment of patients intolerant to TMP-SMX
- If unable to take drug orally with food, consider parenteral administration with an alternative drug
- Drug does NOT provide antimicrobial treatment for concurrent pulmonary infections such as bacterial, viral, or fungal infections
- Follow treatment with secondary prophylaxis (suppression)

PATIENT EDUCATION:
- Take the drug WITH FOOD as directed as food significantly increases absorption of drug
- Take medication for entire 21 days

Azithromycin

BRAND NAME:
- Zithromax

ACTION:
- Broad-spectrum oral antibiotic

INDICATIONS:
- Mild to moderate infections of lower respiratory tract (NOT pneumonia), pharynx/tonsils, skin and skin structures; also, nongonococcal urethritis and cervicitis due to *Chlamydia trachomatis*

CONTRAINDICATIONS:
- Known hypersensitivity to drug, erythromycin, or other macrolide antibiotics
- Use cautiously in renal or hepatic dysfunction
- Pregnancy, nursing mothers

DOSAGE:
- *Adult (≥ 16 years):* 500 mg PO day 1, then 250 mg PO q d days 2–5 (total dose 1.5 gm)
- Nongonococcal urethriitis cervicitis: 1 gm PO X 1

ADMINISTRATION:
- Oral, administer 1 hour before or 2 hours after food

DRUG INTERACTIONS:
- Aluminum- or magnesium-containing antacids: decrease azithromycin absorption, separate by 1–2 hours
- Theophyline: may increase theophylline levels; monitor theophylline levels closely and adjust dose as needed
- Coumadin: may increase prothrombin time (PT); monitor patient closely and adjust coumadin dose as needed

ADVERSE EFFECTS:
- *Uncommon:*
    —Nausea, vomiting, diarrhea, abdominal pain
    —Palpitations, chest pain
    —Vaginitis, monilia superinfection
    —Fatigue, dizziness
    —Rash, photophobia, angioedema
- *Rare:*
    —Pseudomembranous colitis

SPECIAL NURSING CONSIDERATIONS:
- Drug may mask or delay symptoms of gonorrhea and syphilis so patient should have syphilis serology and gonorrheal cultures performed, and treated if results are positive
- Overgrowth of nonsusceptible organisms may occur (e.g., fungi)

PATIENT EDUCATION:
* Take drug 1 hour before or 2 hours after meals
* DO NOT take aluminum or magnesium containing antacids with drug
* Report thrush or vaginal candidiasis

Bleomycin

BRAND NAME:
* Blenoxane

ACTION:
* Antineoplastic antibiotic

INDICATIONS:
* Squamous cell carcinomas
* Lymphomas
* Testicular carcinoma
* Used to treat Kaposi's sarcoma, lymphoma

CONTRAINDICATIONS:
* Known hypersensitivity

DOSAGE:
* Test dose may be ordered (in patients with lymphoma): 1–2 u SC or IV one hour before initial and second doses (1 u = 1 mg)
* Lymphoma: m-BACOD: 4 u/m^2 IV on day 1
* Kaposi's sarcoma: ABV: 10u/m^2 IV every 2 weeks with Adriamycin and vincristine or

Bleomycin: 10–15 u/m^2 IV, IM, or SC every 14
days plus vincristine

ADMINISTRATION:
- Should be administered only by nurses skilled
  in chemotherapy administration
- Use safe chemotherapy handling technique
  (see Appendix I) when mixing, administering
  drug
- SC, IM, IV bolus, continuous IV infusion

DRUG INTERACTIONS:
- Digoxin: may decrease oral bioavailability of
  digoxin: increase digoxin dose as needed
- Phenytoin: may decrease pharmacologic effects
  of phenytoin; assess need to increase
  phenytoin dose

ADVERSE EFFECTS:
- Stomatitis
- Hypersensitivity, including anaphylaxis (rare)
- Pulmonary fibrosis (dose and age related)
- Fever, chills, tumor pain
- Anorexia, weight loss, phlebitis

SPECIAL NURSING CONSIDERATIONS:
- Drug may be used to sclerose pleura to relieve
  pleural effusions caused by tumor or
  pneumothorax caused by HIV-related infection
- Pulmonary function tests should be performed
  baseline and periodically during treatment

- Early signs of pulmonary fibrosis are fine crackles, dyspnea
- Drug should be discontinued if pulmonary diffusion capacity (DLCO) falls below 30–35% of pretreatment normal value; value should be corrected for anemia
- If patient requires surgery, NOTIFY ANESTHE-SIOLOGIST that patient has received drug; inspired oxygen concentration MUST NOT EXCEED THAT OF ROOM AIR
- Anaphylaxis has been reported in ~1% of lymphoma patients; physician may order test dose
- Nonmyelosuppressive

PATIENT EDUCATION:
- Oral hygiene qid after meals
- Self-assess for stomatitis, and report to nurse
- Flaking of skin on fingers, nails can occur
- Report any shortness of breath

Buspirone Hydrochloride

BRAND NAME:
- BuSpar

ACTION:
- Selective anxiolytic agent; modulates midbrain activity through effect on many neurotransmitters

INDICATIONS:
- Management of anxiety disorders
- Short-term relief of anxiety symptoms

CONTRAINDICATIONS:
- Known hypersensitivity
- Pregnancy, nursing mothers
- Use with caution in hepatic, renal dysfunction

DOSAGE:
- *Adult:* 5 mg tid; titrate up 5 mg/day every 2–3 days as needed
- Maximum 60 mg/day
- Dose reduce if renal, hepatic dysfunction

ADMINISTRATION:
- Oral, with or without food
- Patients receiving benzodiazepines, other sedative/hypnotic drugs must be weaned gradually before starting buspirone (NO CROSS-TOLERANCE)

DRUG INTERACTIONS:
- Monamine oxidase inhibitors: increases BP; DO NOT GIVE concurrently
- Haloperidol: increases haloperidol serum levels; avoid concurrent use or decrease haloperidol dose
- Alcohol: increases fatigue, drowsiness, dizziness; avoid if possible
- Other CNS depressants: may increase fatigue, drowsiness, dizziness; use together cautiously

ADVERSE EFFECTS:
* *Uncommon:*
  —Dizziness, drowsiness, headache, fatigue, weakness
  —Nausea, dry mouth, vomiting, diarrhea

SPECIAL NURSING CONSIDERATIONS:
* Selective anxiolytic agent, without sedative or anticonvulsant properties. Does not cause physical or psychological dependence
* Buspirone may be more effective in patients with anxiety-related anger, hostility (cognitive and interpersonal problems), while benzodiazepines may be more effective in managing anxiety-related insomnia, muscle tension (somatic treatment)
* Useful in patients with substance abuse potential and/or who are unable to abstain from alcohol, other CNS depressants while taking anxiolytic medication
* Slow onset, but comparable anxiolytic effect to diazepam

PATIENT EDUCATION:
* Slow onset of action with full effect in 3–4 weeks
* Report any side effects
* Avoid driving a car until after determining drug side effects

Butoconazole Nitrate
2% Cream

BRAND NAME:
• Femstat

ACTION:
• Antifungal agent, structurally similar to
  miconazole; damages fungal membrane and
  metabolism

INDICATIONS:
• Vulvovaginal candidiasis (moniliasis)

CONTRAINDICATIONS:
• Known hypersensitivity to drug or ingredients in
  cream

DOSAGE:
• 1 applicator full (5 gm) q d at bedtime X 3 days;
  continue X 3 days as necessary

ADMINISTRATION:
• Intravaginal cream
• Gently insert using applicator
• Do not interrupt course of treatment (e.g.,
  menses, relief of symptoms)

ADVERSE EFFECTS:
• Rare (2%)
• Vulvovaginal burning, itching, discharge,
  soreness

- Headache
- Itching of fingers
- Urinary frequency

DRUG INTERACTIONS:
- None

SPECIAL NURSING CONSIDERATIONS:
- Centers for Disease Control (CDC) recommends imidazole antifungal agents such as butoconazole, with 3–7 day therapy, for vulvovaginal candidiasis
- Clinical cure rate 75–80%; similar to results with clotrimazole, miconazole therapy

PATIENT EDUCATION:
- Administration technique; do not force applicator in if resistance met, contact nurse, physician
- Complete full course of therapy even if menstruating or symptoms have resolved
- Call physician/nurse if irritation occurs/persists

Capreomycin Sulfate

BRAND NAME:
- Capastat Sulfate

ACTION:
- Antimycobacterial antibiotic

INDICATIONS:
- Used together with at least one other antitubercular agent to treat *Mycobacterium tuberculosis, M. boris, M. kansasii, M. avium*

CONTRAINDICATIONS:
- Use with extreme caution in renal impairment or auditory impairment
- Nursing mothers
- Pregnancy only if benefits outweigh risks

DOSAGE:
- 1 gm IM q d X 60–120 days, then 1 gm 2–3 X/ week (MAX dose 20 mg/kg)
- OR 15–30 mg/kg (max 1 gm) q d adult and child
- Reduce dose if renal impairment

ADMINISTRATION:
- Deep IM into large muscle

DRUG INTERACTIONS:
- Nephrotoxic
- Ototoxic: AVOID aminoglylcoside antibiotics, colistin, polymixin B, vancomycin

ADVERSE EFFECTS:
- Hypersensitivity (urticaria, photosensitivity, rash)
- Nephrotoxicity (tubular necrosis, increased BUN/creatinine, proteinuria, positive casts)
- 8th cranial neuropathy (auditory damage→ hearing loss; vestibular damage→ headache, tinnitus, vertigo)

- Pain, induration, sterile abcess at injection site
- Leukocytosis, leukostasis
- Increased LFTS

SPECIAL NURSING CONSIDERATIONS:
- Monitor BUN/creatinine: if BUN > 30 or other evidence of renal dysfunction, reduce dose
- Monitor LFTs
- Assess hearing loss, tinnitus, headache
- Assess baseline renal, auditory function if at risk
- Monitor serum potassium
- Drug prescribed for tuberculosis only in consultation with physician expert in the management of resistant TB

PATIENT EDUCATION:
- Report rash, hearing loss, headache, vertigo, ringing in ears

Cefamandole

BRAND NAME:
- Mandol

ACTION:
- Cephalosporin antibiotic; active against *H. influenza, Klebsiella, Proteus, Staphylococcus aureus, Streptococcus, E. coli*

INDICATIONS:
- Infections of lower respiratory, urinary and biliary tracts, skin, soft tissues, and septicemia

CONTRAINDICATIONS:
- Known hypersensitivity to drug or other cephalosporins, severe allergic response to penicillins
- Use with caution in patients with renal impairment, colitis, penicillin sensitivity

DOSAGE:
- *Adults:* 500 mg–1 gm q 4–8 hours; severe infections 1–2 gm q 4–6 hours
- Dose is reduced in renal impairment based on creatinine clearance

ADMINISTRATION:
- IM or IV only
- Further dilute in 100 mL and infuse IV over 30 minutes
- Administer deep IM into large muscle mass (for example gluteus maximus)

DRUG INTERACTIONS:
- Probenecid: increased serum concentrations of antibiotic; monitor and decrease dose if needed
- Aminoglycosides, penicillins: may have synergistic antibacterial effect against some organisms
- Nephrotoxic drugs (aminoglycosides, colistin, vancomycin): may increase risk of renal dysfunction; avoid if possible

- Magnesium, calcium: incompatible in IV fluid
- Oral anticoagulants; Aspirin: may increase risk of bleeding
- Alcohol: disulfiram-like reaction (flushing, throbbing headache, dyspnea, nausea, vomiting, diaphoresis, chest pain, palpitation, hyperventilation, tachycardia, hypertension, syncope, weakness, blurred vision) when alcohol ingested within 48–72 hours of cefamandole; does not occur if alcohol ingested prior to first antibiotic dose. If no alcohol prior to first dose, avoid alcohol for 72 hours after last dose

ADVERSE EFFECTS:
- Urticaria, pruritis, rash, fever, chills, exfoliative skin reactions
- Nausea, vomiting, diarrhea
- Rarely, pseudomembranous colitis, dizziness, headache, leukopenia
- Superinfection by nonsusceptible organisms (e.g.,vaginal moniliasis)

SPECIAL NURSING CONSIDERATIONS:
- Rotate IM injection sites as drug can cause pain, induration, sterile abcesses
- Change IV site at least every 48 hours, and assess for signs/symptoms of phlebitis. Apply warm packs prn for comfort
- Be alert for hypersensitivity reactions. If patient develops angioedema (e.g., swollen lips), stop drug. Discuss any rash, pruritis with physician

PATIENT EDUCATION:
- Report rash, itching, swollen lips immediately
- Females report vaginal itching
- Females: perineal hygiene

Cefixime

BRAND NAME:
- Suprax

ACTION:
- Oral cephalosporin antibiotic; active against sensitive gram-negative bacteria, and staphlococci

INDICATIONS:
- Uncomplicated urinary tract infections, otitis media, respiratory tract infections
- Used to treat uncomplicated gonorrhea

CONTRAINDICATIONS:
- Known hypersensitivity to drug or other cephalosporin antibiotics, severe hypersensitivity to penicillins, pregnant or nursing mothers
- Use cautiously in patients with renal dysfunction, colitis

DOSAGE:
- *Adults:* 400 mg PO daily (in 1 or 2 divided doses q 12 hours) X 5–10 days (UTI, URI), or 10–14 days (lower respiratory tract)

- Children (> 12 years & > 50 kg): adult dose
- Children (6 months–12 years): 8 mg/kg/day in single or 2 divided doses q 12 hours
- Reduce dose if urine creatinine clearance < 60 mL/minute

ADMINISTRATION:
- Oral, without meals

DRUG INTERACTIONS:
- Probenecid: increases serum concentrations of antibiotic; used in combination to advantage

ADVERSE EFFECTS:
- *Usually mild:*
  —Diarrhea or loose stools, abdominal pain, nausea, vomiting
  —Urticaria, rash, pruritis, arthralgia
- *Rare:*
  —Pseudomembranous colitis, leukopenia, thrombocytopenia
  —Headache, nervousness, insomnia
  —Transient, increased liver function and renal function tests

SPECIAL NURSING CONSIDERATIONS:
- Superinfection of nonsusceptible organisms can occur

PATIENT EDUCATION:
- Report rash immediately
- Take drug with meals if gastric upset occurs
- Females: report vaginal itch

Cefoxitin

BRAND NAME:
- Mefoxin

ACTION:
- Cephalosporin antibiotic; active against sensitive gram-negative and some gram-positive bacteria

INDICATIONS:
- Infections caused by sensitive organisms in upper and lower respiratory tract, urinary tract, skin, and pelvis
- Used in treatment of uncomplicated gonorrhea; second-line, not recommended by Centers for Disease Control (CDC)

CONTRAINDICATIONS:
- Known hypersensitivity to drug, other cephalosporin or penicillin antibiotics
- Use cautiously in patients with history of colitis

DOSAGE:
- *Adult:* 1–2 gm q 6–8 hours (max 12 gm/24 hours in divided doses)
- *Children:* (3 months or older): 80–160 mg/kg/day in 3–6 equally divided doses
- Dose reduce in renal dysfunction based on creatinine clearance

ADMINISTRATION:
- IV: further dilute reconstituted solution and administer over 30–60 minutes
- IM: deep IM in large muscle mass

DRUG INTERACTIONS:
- Probenecid: increased serum concentration of antibiotic; monitor and decrease dose if needed
- Aminoglycosides, penicillins: may have synergistic antibacterial effect against some organisms
- Nephrotoxic drugs (aminoglycosides, colistin, vancomycin): may increase risk of renal dysfunction; avoid if possible
- Magnesium, calcium: incompatible in IV fluid
- Oral anticoagulants; Aspirin: may increase risk of bleeding
- Alcohol: disulfiram-like reaction (flushing, throbbing headache, dyspnea, nausea, vomiting, diaphoresis, chest pain, palpitation, hyperventilation, tachycardia, hypertension, syncope, weakness, blurred vision) when alcohol ingested prior to first antibiotic dose. Avoid alcohol prior to first dose during treatment, and for 72 hours after last dose

ADVERSE EFFECTS:
- Rash, pruritis, urticaria, fever
- Pain, induration, tenderness after IM injection
- Thrombophlebitis after IV injection

- Rarely, transient increase in renal function tests, leukopenia, thrombocytopenia, nausea, vomiting, pseudomembranous colitis

SPECIAL NURSING CONSIDERATIONS:
- Treatment for gonorrhea should be followed by oral doxycycline, or tetracycline or erythromycin therapy to treat chlamydia in heterosexual men (homosexual men are NOT likely to have coexisting chlamydial infection)
- Discontinue drug if hypertensivity occurs
- IM discomfort can be decreased by using 0.5% or 1% lidocaine hydrochloride (without epineph-rine) as drug diluent
- IV discomfort can be decreased by using butterfly or scalp vein needle sets rather than polyethylene catheters

PATIENT EDUCATION:
- Report rash, itching immediately
- Avoid alchohol before, during, and for 72 hours after treatment

Ceftriaxone Sodium

BRAND NAME:
- Rocephin

ACTION:
- Cephalosporin antibiotic; active against gram-negative cocci and some gram-positive bacteria

INDICATIONS:
- Infections of lower respiratory and urinary tracts, skin, bone and joint, abdomen, as well as meningitis and sepsis
- Gonorrhea caused by penicillinase-producing *N. gonorrhoeae* (PPNG)

CONTRAINDICATIONS:
- Known hypersensitivity to drug, other cephalosporins
- Severe hypersensitivity to penicillin antibiotics
- Use cautiously if history of colitis, gallbladder disease

DOSAGE:
- *Adult, children ≥ 12 years:* 1–2 gm q d or in equally divided doses q 12 hours doses; CNS infections may require 4 gm/day in divided doses
- *Adult* (uncomplicated gonorrhea): single 250 mg dose IM

ADMINISTRATION:
- IM: give deep IM in large muscle mass (e.g., gluteus maximus)
- IV: infuse further diluted drug over 30–60 minutes

DRUG INTERACTIONS:
- Aminoglycosides, penicillins: possible synergism

- Nephrotoxic drugs (aminoglycosides, colistin, vancomycin): increase risk of nephrotoxicity, use cautiously and monitor renal function closely
- Probenecid: increases serum antibiotic levels; use together to advantage

ADVERSE EFFECTS:
- Pain, induration, tenderness at injection site
- *Uncommon:*
  —Urticaria, pruritis, rash, fever, chills, myalgias
  —Eosinophilia, leukopenia
  —Diarrhea, nausea, vomiting, dysgeusia
  —Increased liver and renal function tests
  —Superinfection by nonsusceptible organisms (e.g., candidiasis)

SPECIAL NURSING CONSIDERATIONS:
- Drug has been used in the treatment of syphillis
- IM: manufacturer states 1% lidocaine HCl (without epinephrine) can be used as diluent to decrease injection pain
- Discontinue drug if symptoms of gallbladder inflammation occur (drug may precipitate in gallbladder) or if rash develops
- Monitor CBC, liver and renal function tests, baseline and periodically during extended treatment
- Drug of choice for PPNG gonorrhea

- When drug given for uncomplicated gonorrhea, drug should be followed by oral doxycycline, tetracycline, or erythromycin therapy to eradicate coexisting *Chlamydia* infection

PATIENT EDUCATION:
- Report rash immediately
- Report gastrointestinal symptoms
- Report thrush, or vaginal itching (females)

Cefuroxime Axetil (Oral)
Cefuroxime Sodium
(Parenteral)

BRAND NAMES:
- (Oral): Ceftin
  (Parenteral): Kefurox, Zinacef

ACTION:
- Synthetic cephalosporin antibiotic; active against gram-negative organisms, including many that produce beta-lactamase

INDICATIONS:
- Orally to treat infections of lower respiratory and urinary tracts, pharynx, skin, and skin structures

- Parenterally, to treat serious infections of lower respiratory and urinary tracts, pharynx, skin, bone and joint, as well as septicemia and meningitis
- Used to treat uncomplicated gonorrhea or disseminated infections

CONTRAINDICATIONS:
- Known hypersensitivity to drug, other cephalosporins, or penicillin antibiotics
- Use with caution in patients with history of colitis, or in pregnancy or nursing mothers

DOSAGE:
- Oral:
  —*Adults:* 250–500 mg q 12 hours
  —*Children: (2–12 years)*: 125–250 mg q 12 hours
- *Parenteral:*
  —Adults: 750 mg–1.5 gm q 8 hours;
  —Gonorrhea: single 1.5 gm dose IM plus 1 gm oral probenecid
- Decrease dose in renal dysfunction

ADMINISTRATION:
- Cefuroxime axetil (oral): give with meals if possible
- Cefuroxime sodium (parenteral):
  —IV: infuse over 15–60 minutes
  —IM: give deep into large muscle mass
  —Gonorrhea: 1.5 gm dose should be divided and given in two sites

DRUG INTERACTIONS:
- Probenecid: increases serum antibiotic levels; use in combination to advantage
- Aminoglycoside antibiotics: additive or synergistic action against some organisms, with increased risk of renal toxicity; use to advantage but monitor renal function
- Diuretics: possible increase in nephrotoxicity; monitor renal function closely

ADVERSE EFFECTS:
- Local reactions at injection site
- Thrombophlebitis
- *Uncommon:*
  —Rash, fever, urticaria, pruritis
  —Nausea, vomiting, diarrhea
  —Pseudomembranous colitis
  —Decreased hemoglobin/hematocrit, transient neutropenia
  —Transient increase in liver and renal function tests
  —Headache, dizziness
  —Superinfection by nonsusceptible organisms (e.g., vaginal candidiasis)

SPECIAL NURSING CONSIDERATIONS:
- Assess for signs/symptoms of fungal superinfection (oral, perirectal, vaginal)
- Assess renal function baseline and periodically during treatment, especially with high doses in seriously ill patients

PATIENT EDUCATION:
- Report rash immediately
- Report thrush, perianal, or vaginal candidiasis

Chloral Hydrate

BRAND NAMES:
- Noctec, Aquachloral supprettes

ACTION:
- Sedative, hypnotic agent; produces quiet, deep sleep

INDICATIONS:
- Short-term treatment of insomnia

CONTRAINDICATIONS:
- Known hypersensitivity, severe hepatic or renal dysfunction
- Use with caution, if at all, in severe cardiac disease, mental depression, suicidal ideation, history of drug abuse, pregnancy, nursing mothers

DOSAGE:
- *Adults:* 500 mg–1 gm PO/PR 30 minutes before HS (max dose 2 gm)
- *Children:* 50 mg/kg or 1.5 gm/m^2 (max 1 gm) 30 minutes before HS

ADMINISTRATION:
- Oral: give with full glass of liquid; oral solution should be well diluted. Do not administer oral dosage to patients with gastritis, esophagitis, or ulcers
- Rectal: suppository or retention enema

DRUG INTERACTIONS:
- CNS depressants (alcohol, barbiturates): increase CNS depression; AVOID concurrent use
- Coumadin: may increase prothrombin time (PT); monitor PT closely

ADVERSE EFFECTS:
- Nausea, vomiting, diarrhea
- Residual sedation, "hangover"
- Tolerance, physical and psychological dependence may develop when used for ≥ 2 weeks
- *Uncommon:*
  —Rash
  —Leukopenia, eosinophilia

SPECIAL NURSING CONSIDERATIONS:
- Assess for signs/symptoms of drug dependency:
  —Drowsiness, lethargy, nystagmus, tremulousness, lack of coordination, slurred speech
- Drug should be withdrawn gradually when used chronically to prevent withdrawal symptoms

- Drug may impair ability to drive a car
- Avoid concurrent alcohol use
- Take medication as instructed

Chlorhexadine Gluconate Oral Rinse

BRAND NAME:
- Peridex

ACTION:
- Antimicrobial oral rinse, contains 0.12% chlorhexidine gluconate; significantly reduces gingivitis as well as oral infections after chemotherapy

INDICATIONS:
- Gingivitis
- Used to prevent oral infections in immunosuppressed patients receiving cancer chemotherapy

CONTRAINDICATIONS:
- Known hypersensitivity

DOSAGE:
- 15 mL oral rinse for 30 seconds bid

ADMINISTRATION:
- Oral rinse, in morning and evening after brushing teeth

DRUG INTERACTIONS:
- None known

ADVERSE EFFECTS:
- Staining of teeth, oral surfaces in some patients
- Increased supragingival calculus formation
- Altered taste perception

SPECIAL NURSING CONSIDERATIONS:
- Drug is blue solution
- Treatment should begin after oral dental prophylaxis, although this is not always feasible

PATIENT EDUCATION:
- Some patients may develop stained teeth
- Taste may become altered
- Use oral rinse after brushing teeth (soft tooth-brush) in morning and evening

Clarithromycin

BRAND NAME:
- Biaxin

ACTION:
- Broad-spectrum oral antibiotic

INDICATIONS:
- Mild to moderate infections of upper respiratory tract (including pneumonia due to *Mycoplasma*), and uncomplicated skin and skin structures

CONTRAINDICATIONS:
- Known hypersensitivity to drug, erythromycin, or other macrolide antibiotics
- Pregnancy, nursing mothers

DOSAGE:
- Adults: upper respiratory tract infections: 250–500 mg q 12 hours X 10–14 days
- Adults: lower respiratory tract infections: 250–500 mg q 12 hours X 7–14 days
- Adults: skin infections: 250 mg q 12 hours X 7–14 days
- Dose may be reduced in renal failure

ADMINISTRATION:
- Oral, take without regard to meals

DRUG INTERACTIONS:
- Theophylline: increases serum theophylline level; monitor serum levels and decrease theophylline dose

ADVERSE EFFECTS:
- *Uncommon:*
  —Diarrhea
  —Nausea, abnormal taste, dyspepsia

—Abdominal pain, discomfort
—Headache
- *Rare:*
—Pseudomembranous colitis

SPECIAL NURSING CONSIDERATIONS:
- Drug is used experimentally alone or in combination with other drugs to prevent *Mycobacterium avium* complex (MAC)

PATIENT EDUCATION:
- Take without regard to meals

Ciprofloxacin

BRAND NAME:
- Cipro

ACTION:
- Quinolone antibiotic; broad-spectrum activity against most gram-negative and some gram-positive organisms

INDICATIONS:
- Infections of lower respiratory, gastrointestinal, and urinary tracts; skin, bone and joint. Also used to treat gonorrhea

CONTRAINDICATIONS:
- Known hypersensitivity to drug or other quinolone antibiotics

- Pregnant or nursing mothers
- Use cautiously in patients with seizure disorders or who are receiving theophylline

DOSAGE:
- *Adults:* oral: 250–750 mg q 12 hours depending on site of infections X 1–2 weeks
- IV: 200–400 mg q 12 hours X 1–2 weeks (if unable to take oral)
- Dose reduce in renal dysfunction based on creatinine clearance

ADMINISTRATION:
- Oral route preferred; take with 1 large glass of fluid, 2 hours after meal/food
- IV: if unable to take orally; infuse over 60 minutes
- Optimal peak concentrations (1–2 hours after dosing) are 2–4 µg/mL

DRUG INTERACTIONS:
- Antacids (containing magnesium, aluminum, or calcium): decreases oral ciprofloxacin serum level; do not administer concurrently. If must administer antacids, administer at least 2 hours apart
- Other anti-infectives: potential synergism with clindamycin, aminoglycosides, beta-lactam antibiotics against certain organisms
- Probenecid: 50% increase in ciprofloxacin serum levels; decrease ciprofloxacin dose if given concurrently

- Theophylline: increases theophylline serum level; avoid if possible since fatal reactions have occurred. Otherwise, monitor theophylline level very closely and decrease theophylline dose as needed.
- Caffeine: delays caffeine clearance from body. Teach patient to limit coffee, tea, soft drinks, especially if CNS side effects.

ADVERSE EFFECTS:
- Nausea, vomiting, abdominal discomfort, diarrhea, anorexia
- Superinfection of nonsusceptible organisms (fungi)
- Local reaction at IV site (pain, inflammation)
- Photosensitivity
- *Uncommon:*
    —Headache, restlessness
    —Increased BUN, serum creatinine
    —Rash, eosinophilia, fever, chills, anaphylaxis

SPECIAL NURSING CONSIDERATIONS:
- Monitor BUN, serum creatinine baseline and periodically during treatment
- Apply heat to IV site as needed to promote comfort
- Assess for signs/symptoms of candidiasis on mucous membranes
- When drug used as second line to treat resistant TB, drug should be prescribed in consultation with a physician expert in the management of resistant TB

PATIENT EDUCATION:
- Reduce caffeine intake
- Avoid prolonged direct sunlight; use sunblock (skin protection factor 15)
- Increase oral fluid intake to 2–3 quarts/day
- Females: report vaginal itching, burning

Clindamycin Hydrochloride

BRAND NAME:
- Cleocin

ACTION:
- Lincosamine antibiotic, active against most aerobic gram-positive cocci and some anaerobic gram-positive and gram-negative organisms. Also active against *Mycoplasma* and *Neisseria* gonorrhea.

INDICATIONS:
- Serious infections of respiratory and female pelvic/genital tract, skin/soft tissues
- Used investigationally with other drugs in treatment of *Mycobacterium avium* complex (MAC); may also be used to treat *Pneumocystis carinii* pneumonia (PCP) with primaquine and to treat cryptosporidiosis and toxoplasmosis in AIDS patients

CONTRAINDICATIONS:
- Hypersensitivity to clindamycin or lincomycin
- History of colitis
- Pregnancy or nursing mothers

DOSAGE:
- *Adult:* oral: 150–450 mg PO q 6 hours; IM/IV: 300 mg q 6–12 hours (MAX 2.7 gm/day)
- *Children:* (> 10 kg): 8–25 mg/kg/day in 3 or 4 equally divided doses

ADMINISTRATION:
- Administer orally with 8 oz. of water
- IM dose should not exceed 600 mg
- IV dose should not exceed 1.2 gm in 1 hour period, and infuse over 30–60 minutes. May give as continuous infusion
- DO NOT GIVE RAPID BOLUS

DRUG INTERACTIONS:
- Neuromuscular blocking agents (tubocurarine, ether, pancuronium); may increase neuromuscular blockade; use concurrently with caution
- Erythromycin: decreases bactericidal activity or clindamycin
- Kaolin: decreases GI absorption of clindamycin. Avoid concurrent administration, or administer at least 2 hours apart

ADVERSE EFFECTS:
- Nausea, vomiting, diarrhea, abdominal pain, tenesmus

- Maculopapular rash, urticaria
- Local discomfort at injection site (IM or IV)
- Rare: fatal pseudomembranous colitis (severe diarrhea, abdominal cramping, melena, beginning 2–9 days after drug initiated).

SPECIAL NURSING CONSIDERATIONS:
- Can cause fatal colitis: stop drug if diarrhea occurs, or, if necessary, continue only with close monitoring and endoscopy
- Apply heat to reduce local discomfort

PATIENT EDUCATION:
- Take drug with 8 oz. of water
- Stop drug and report diarrhea, rash, immediately

Clofazimine

BRAND NAME:
- Lamprene

ACTION:
- Phenazine dye with antimycobacterial and anti-inflammatory actions

INDICATIONS:
- Leprosy (used with at least one other drug)
- Used investigationally in treatment of *Mycobacterium avium* intracellular (MAI) infections in patients with HIV

CONTRAINDICATIONS:
- None
- Use with extreme caution in patients with abdominal pain and diarrhea

DOSAGE:
- MAI: *adults:* 100 mg PO 1 or 3 X daily
- Leprosy: 50–100 mg q d

ADMINISTRATION:
- Orally, with meals

DRUG INTERACTIONS:
- Rifampin: decreases absorption of rifampin
- Isoniazid: increases clofazimine serum levels and decreases drug concentration in skin

ADVERSE EFFECTS:
- Pink to brownish bronze skin discoloration
- Dry skin
- Reversible red-brown discoloration of conjunctiva, cornea, lacrimal fluid
- Abdominal and epigastric pain, diarrhea, nausea, vomiting
- Rarely, splenic infarction, bowel obstruction

SPECIAL NURSING CONSIDERATIONS:
- Drug used off-label and not approved by U.S. Food and Drug Administration for MAI infections
- One multidrug regime used includes rifabutin, clofazimine, isoniazid, and ethambutol

- No regime clearly effective for treatment of MAI (now called MAC, *Mycobacterium avium* complex) in patients with HIV, and many clinical trials underway
- Skin discoloration may lead to depression; 2 suicides have been reported
- Drug dose should be decreased (or drug discontinued if severe) if patient developes colic, burning abdominal pain, nausea/vomiting, diarrhea as splenic infarction, bowel obstruction, and GI bleeding may occur

PATIENT EDUCATION:
- Drug may cause reversible pink to brownish-black discoloration of skin, conjunctiva, sweat, urine, feces
- Report depression or changes in feeling state to nurse or physician
- Report colic, or burning abdominal pain, nausea, vomiting, diarrhea immediately

Clotrimazole

BRAND NAMES:
- Mycelex Troche (oral use)
- Mycelex-G vaginal tablet
- Lotrimin cream, lotion, solution
- Gyne-Lotrimin vaginal cream

ACTION:
- Antifungal agent. Binds to fungal cell membrane, altering permeability and causes cell death

INDICATIONS:
- Oropharyngeal candidiasis
- Dermatophytoses, superficial mycoses, cutaneous candidiasis
- Vulvovaginal candidiasis (moniliasis)

CONTRAINDICATIONS:
- Hypersensitivity to drug or ingredients

DOSAGE:
- *Adult:*
  —Oral (oropharyngeal): 10 mg lozenge 5 times/day X 14 days
  —Vaginal: 2 vaginal tablets containing 100 mg each (total 200 mg) intravaginally q d X 3–7 days; or 1 applicator full of cream (5 grams) q d X 7–14 days
  —Topical: apply 1% cream, 1% lotion, or 1% solution sparingly to affected area X 1–8 weeks

ADMINISTRATION:
- Oral: slowly dissolve tablet in mouth for 15–30 minutes
- Vaginal: insert tablets or applicatorful of vaginal cream at bedtime

DRUG INTERACTIONS:
- None known

ADVERSE EFFECTS:
- Skin blistering, erythema, pruritis, burning, urticaria
- Occasional vaginal irritation, slight cramping, dyspareunia (vaginal tablets or creams)
- Transient increase in liver function tests (AST), nausea, vomiting (lozenges)

SPECIAL NURSING CONSIDERATIONS:
- Monitor liver function tests baseline and periodically during treatment with oral lozenges, especially in patients with hepatic dysfunction

PATIENT EDUCATION:
- Dissolve lozenges slowly in mouth
- Do not use vaginal tampons when using vaginal tablets or cream

Codeine (Phosphate or Sulfate)

BRAND NAME:
- Codeine

ACTION:
- Narcotic analgesic; useful for mild to moderate pain unrelieved by nonnarcotic analgesics

INDICATIONS:
- Mild to moderate pain

CONTRAINDICATIONS:
- Known hypersensitivity
- Use with caution in hepatic or renal impairment, hypothyroidism
- Severe CNS depression, respiratory depression, head injury

DOSAGE:
- *Adult:* 30 mg q 4 hours (range 15 mg–60 mg), PO, SC, IM
- *Children:* 3 mg/kg or 100 mg/m^2 daily in 6 divided doses

ADMINISTRATION:
- Oral, SC, IM

DRUG INTERACTIONS:
- Injection incompatible with solutions containing aminophylline, ammonium chloride, amobarbital sodium, chlorothiazide sodium, heparin sodium, methicillin sodium, nitrofurantoin, phenobarbital sodium, sodium bicarbonate
- Alcohol, CNS depressants: additive effects
- Acetaminophen, aspirin: additive analgesia; use together to advantage

ADVERSE EFFECTS:
- Psychological dependence
- Drowsiness, sedation, mood changes, dizziness
- Constipation

- Nausea, vomiting, dry mouth
- Orthostatic hypotension, bradycardia
- Urinary urgency, retention, dysuria

SPECIAL NURSING CONSIDERATIONS:
- Combination preparations:
  —Codeine plus acetaminophen 300 mg: Tylenol with codeine No.1 (Codeine 7.5 mg/ acetaminophen 300 mg); No. 2 (Codeine 15 mg); No. 3 (Codeine 30 mg); No. 4 (Codeine 60 mg)
  —Codeine plus aspirin 325 mg: empirin with codeine 15 mg (No. 2), Empirin with codeine 30 mg (No. 3), Empirin with codeine 60 mg (No. 4)
- Parenteral dose is two-thirds oral dose (equianalgesic dose)
- Onset of action after oral or subcutaneous dose is 15–30 minutes with duration of 4–6 hours
- Give smallest effective dose to prevent tolerance, physical dependency

PATIENT EDUCATION:
- Daily bowel regime (high fiber diet, fluids to 3 L/ day, exercise as tolerated) to ensure bowel movement at least every other day
- Take only when needed to prevent or relieve pain

Cyclophosphamide

BRAND NAMES:
- Cytoxan, Neosar

ACTION:
- Alkylating, antineoplastic agent; causes cross-linking of DNA strands preventing DNA synthesis

INDICATIONS:
- Non-Hodgkin's lymphoma
- Hodgkin's disease

CONTRAINDICATIONS:
- Known hypersensitivity
- Neutropenia, thrombocytopenia

DOSAGE:
- HIV Lymphoma:
  - —m-BACOD: usal dosage
    - –Cyclophosphamide 600 mg/m^2 IV day 1 repeated q 3 weeks
    - –Plus G-CSF (Filgrastim) or GM-CSF (Sargramostim)
  - —m-BACOD: modified dosage
    - –300 mg/m^2 IV day 1 repeated q 3 weeks
  - —CHOP: modified dosage
    - –400–500 mg/m^2 IV day 1

ADMINISTRATION:
- IV: ensure patient well hydrated; administer IV over 20–60 minutes
- Also available in oral tablets
- Should only be administered by nurses skilled in the administration of chemotherapy treatment
- USE SAFE CHEMOTHERAPY HANDLING PRECAUTIONS (see Appendix I)

DRUG INTERACTIONS:
- Increases chloramphenicol half-life
- Increases duration of leukopenia when given in combination with thiazide diuretics
- Increases effect of anticoagulant drugs
- Decreases digoxin level so dose may need to be increased
- Potentiates doxorubicin-induced cardiomyopathy at high doses
- Increases succinylcholine action with prolonged neuromuscular blockage
- Increases drug action of barbiturates; causes induction of hepatic microsomes

ADVERSE EFFECTS:
- Nausea/vomiting, anorexia
- Hemorrhagic cystitis if drug metabolites permitted to accumulate in bladder
- Neutropenia (nadir, day 7–14, recovery in 1–2 weeks)
- Immunosuppression

- Alopecia (temporary), hyperpigmentation of nails, skin
- Reproductive alterations: amenorrhea, oligospermia

SPECIAL NURSING CONSIDERATIONS:
- m-BACOD: methotrexate, Leukovorin, Bleomycin, Doxorubicin, Cyclophosphamide, Vincristine, Dexamethasone
- Ensure patient well hydrated pre- and postadministration. Encourage patient to void q 2–3 hours to prevent hemorrhagic cystitis
- Premedicate with antiemetic(s) prior to dose, and continue for 24 hours, at least for initial dose

PATIENT EDUCATION:
- Avoid aspirin
- Notify physician, nurse if fever (unusual) or bleeding occur
- Increase PO intake to 3 L/day X 3 days
- Void q 2–3 hours
- Hair will grow back after treatment
- Nails may become hyperpigmented

Cycloserine

BRAND NAME:
- Seromycin Pulvules

ACTION:
- Antimycobacterial antibiotic; inhibits bacterial cell wall synthesis

INDICATIONS:
- Active pulmonary and extrapulmonary tuberculosis, caused by susceptible mycobacteria unresponsive to first-line therapy (e.g., streptomycin, isoniazid, rifampin, ethambutol)
- Used as adjunct with other drugs

CONTRAINDICATIONS:
- Pregnancy, nursing mothers unless benefit outweighs risk
- Concurrent alcohol abuse
- Known hypersensitivity
- Epilepsy
- Depression, severe anxiety, psychosis
- Renal insufficiency/failure

DOSAGE:
- *Adults:* 250 mg PO q 12 hours X 12 weeks, then dose titrated to maintain serum level < 30 µg/mL (usually 0.5–1 gm q d *in divided doses*)
- Modify dose +/or frequency of administration if renal dysfunction exists

ADMINISTRATION:
- Orally
- Available as 250 mg tablets

DRUG INTERACTIONS:
- Ethionamide: increased neeurotoxicity; avoid concurrent use
- Alcohol: increased risk of epileptic seizures; DO NOT COMBINE
- Isoniazid: may increase risk of CNS toxicity; monitor closely
- Phenytoin: increased serum levels; monitor for phenytoin toxicity and dose reduce as needed

ADVERSE EFFECTS:
- CNS toxicity (increase risk with doses > 500 mg) : dizziness, drowsiness, lethargy, sedation, depression, tremor, dysarthria, paresthesia, confusion, memory loss, seizures
- Hypersensitivity (rash, photosensitivity)
- Rarely, anemia

SPECIAL NURSING CONSIDERATIONS:
- Monitor baseline and periodic renal, hepatic function studies, and CBC
- Monitor serum cycloserine concentrations at least weekly if drug dose > 500 mg daily
- Assess and monitor closely for signs/symptoms of CNS toxicity, especially during first 2 weeks of therapy. If signs/symptoms occur, drug dose should be reduced, then discontinued if signs/symptoms DO NOT RESOLVE
- Neurotoxicity may be reduced/ prevented with pyridoxine 200 mg–300 mg PO daily

- When drug used as second line to treat resistant TB, drug should be prescribed in consultation with a physician expert in the management of resistant TB

PATIENT EDUCATION:
- Do not drink alcohol while taking drug
- Assess for and report signs/symptoms of dizziness, sedation, depression, mental changes, paresthesia.
- If seizures occur, stop drug; call physician immediately or come to emergency room

Cytarabine, Cytosine Arabinosine

BRAND NAMES:
- Arabinosyl Cytosine, Ara-C, Cytarabine Cytosar-U

ACTION:
- Antimetabolite antineoplastic agent; interferes with synthesis of DNA, causing cell death

INDICATIONS:
- Leukemia
- Used in treatment of meningeal lymphoma (e.g., HIV lymphoma)

CONTRAINDICATIONS:
- Known hypersensitivity
- Neutropenia, thrombocytopenia unless tumor-related

DOSAGE:
- Leukemia: 100 mg/m^2 IV continuous infusion X 5–10 days with daunorubicin
- Intrathecal (IT): 20–30 mg/m^2 q d X 4–5 days, but varies with whether drug is given for CNS prophylaxis (e.g., 50 mg IT q week X 4) or treatment of lymphomatous meningitis 50 mg IT 3 X/week until CSF cytology clear, then q week
- Reduce dose in hepatic impairment

ADMINISTRATION:
- IV: as continuous infusion (leukemia) or IV bolus (lymphoma)
- IT: preservative-free diluent, and sterile technique must be used
- Drug should only be administered by a nurse skilled in chemotherapy administration
- USE SAFE CHEMOTHERAPY HANDLING PRECAUTIONS (see Appendix I)

DRUG INTERACTIONS:
- Digoxin may decrease bioavailability of digoxin; monitor serum digoxin level
- Bone marrow suppressive agents: increase bone marrow depression

ADVERSE EFFECTS:

- IT: nausea, vomiting, fever, transient head-aches; rarely, paresthesia, paraplegia, spastic paraparesis
- IV:
  —Neutropenia (nadir 7–9 days)
  —Thrombocytopenia (nadir, day 12–15)
  —Nausea, anemia, vomiting, anorexia, stomatitis
  —Hepatotoxicity
  —Rash, alopecia
  —Neurotoxicity at high doses
  —Tumor lysis syndrome (induction therapy in leukemia) with increased uric acid, potassium, phosphorus, BUN, serum creatinine

SPECIAL NURSING CONSIDERATIONS:

- Give antiemetic prior to systemic therapy
- Monitor CBC, absolute neutrophil count baseline and frequently during treatment
- Even when drug given IT, drug leaks into systemic circulation, and may cause bone marrow suppression
- Induction therapy for leukemia; ensure adequate hydration, alkalinization of urine, and allopurinol to reduce risk of tumor lysis syndrome

PATIENT EDUCATION:
- Notify physician, nurse if fever, bleeding occur
- Avoid aspirin, aspirin-containing drugs, NSAIDs
- Use regular oral hygiene; notify nurse if stomatitis develops

Dapsone

BRAND NAME:
- Dapsone

ACTION:
- Antibacterial against *Mycobacterium leprae*

INDICATIONS:
- Leprosy, dermatitis herpetiformis
- Used second-line for treatment or prophylaxis of *Pneumocystis carinii* pneumonia (PCP)

CONTRAINDICATIONS:
- Hypersensitivity to drug
- Patients with glucose-6-phosphate dehydrogenase (G6PD) deficiency, or severe anemia
- Use cautiously in pregnancy

DOSAGE:
- PCP: Dapsone 100 mg PO X 21 days; trimethoprim (20 mg/kg daily in 4 divided doses) may be added
- PCP prophylaxsis: Dapsone 50–100 mg PO q d to 3 X/wk

ADMINISTRATION:
- Oral

DRUG INTERACTIONS:
- Rifampin: decreases dapsone serum levels seven-to tenfold; may need to increase dapsone dose
- Folinic acid antagonists (pyrimethamine, methotrexate): increases hematologic toxicity; avoid concurrent use
- Didanosine: buffer decreases dapsone absorption; administer 2 hours apart

ADVERSE EFFECTS:
- Hemolysis of red blood cells with anemia; methemoglobinemia (combined dapsone, trimethoprim)
- Peripheral neuropathy (rare)
- Nausea, vomiting, abdominal pain
- Headache, abnormal liver function tests
- Rash (30–40% incidence in AIDS patients receiving dapsone/trimethoprim)
- Vertigo, blurred vision, insomnia

SPECIAL NURSING CONSIDERATIONS:
- In treatment of initial episodes of PCP, dapsone and trimethoprim are as effective as oral co-trimoxazole and better tolerated
- Screen HIV patients for G6PD deficiency

- Monitor weekly hemoglobin, methemoglobin concentrations and hematocrit in patients receiving dapsone/trimethoprim
- Monitor baseline and periodic liver function tests

PATIENT EDUCATION:
- Report fever, chills, jaundice, purpura immediately
- Report rash immediately to determine drug continuance

Dexamethasone

BRAND NAME:
- Decadron

ACTION:
- Glucocorticoid steroid; causes destruction of lymphoid malignant cells, reduces cerebral edema, and decreases nausea/vomiting following cancer chemotherapy

INDICATIONS:
- Lymphoma, leukemia, increased cerebral edema
- Used as antiemetic in combination with other agents

CONTRAINDICATIONS:
- Known hypersensitivity, psychosis, idiopathic thrombocytopenia, amebiasis, fungal infections, acute glomerulonephritis

DOSAGE:
- Treatment of lymphoma (m-BACO*D*): 6 mg/m^2 orally days 1–5 q 21 days
- Cerebral edema: 10 mg IV then 4 mg q 6 hours until symptoms subside, or other treatment initiated (e.g., radiotherapy)
- Antiemetic: 10–20 mg IV prior to chemotherapy

ADMINISTRATION:
- Oral: administer with food or milk
- IV: may be given with H$_2$ antagonist to prevent gastric irritation

DRUG INTERACTIONS:
- Indomethacin, aspirin: increases GI irritation and bleeding; avoid concurrent use
- Barbiturates, phenytoin, rifampin: decreases dexamethasone effect; increase dose as needed

ADVERSE EFFECTS:
- Increases appetite, abdominal distention, GI hemorrhage
- Euphoria, mood swings, depression, cataracts
- Congestive heart failure, fluid retention, hypertension
- Hyperglycemia, hypokalemia

SPECIAL NURSING CONSIDERATIONS:
- If patient receives dexamethasone chronically, drug must be tapered to prevent withdrawal
- m-BACOD: Methotrexate, Bleomycin, Adriamycin, Cytoxan, Oncovin, Dexamethasone combination chemotherapy for lymphoma
- Monitor blood glucose closely if patient has diabetes or carbohydrate intolerance
- Assess BP, weight, and evidence of edema

PATIENT EDUCATION:
- Take drug with food or milk
- Report signs/symptoms of hyperglycemia, especially if taking drug for extended period

Didanosine (ddl)

BRAND NAME:
- Videx

ACTION:
- Antiretroviral agent; nucleoside analogue that inhibits the enzyme reverse transcription, thus preventing viral replication

INDICATIONS:
- Management of advanced HIV disease in adults and children over 6 months who are unable to tolerate zidovudine therapy, or who show

obvious clinical or immunologic deterioration
on zidovudine

CONTRAINDICATIONS:
- Known hypersensitivity to drug or its ingredients
- Pregnant or breast-feeding women
- Use cautiously, if at all, in patients with a history of pancreatitis or with risk factors (increased amylase, increased triglycerides, alcohol abuse)
- Use cautiously, if at all, in patients with a history of peripheral neuropathy

DOSAGE (by weight):
- *Adult:* **chewable, dispersible buffered tablet** (each dose should be at least 2 tablets to ensure adequate buffering): 200 mg q 12 hours, weight ≥ 50 kg; 125 mg q 12 hours, weight < 50 kg; **oral solution prepared from buffered powder:** 250 mg q 12 hours, weight ≥ 50 kg; 167 mg q 12 hours, weight < 50 kg
- *Children:* age > 1 year, dose should be at least 2 tablets; < 1 year of age, 1 tablet; **chewable, buffered dispersible tablet** (by body surface area or BSA): BSA 1.1–1.4 m^2 = 100 mg q 12 hours; 0.8–1.0 m^2 = 75 mg q 12 hours; 0.5–0.7 m^2 = 50 mg q 12 hours; < 0.5 m^2= 25 mg q 12 hours; **reconstituted pediatric oral solution** (10 mg/ mL): BSA 1.1–1.4m^2 = 125mg (12.5 mL) q 12 hours; 0.8–1.0m^2 = 94 mg (9.5 mL) q 12 hours; 0.5–0.7m^2 = 62 mg (6 mL) q 12 hours; < 0.5 m^2 = 31 mg (3 mL) q 12 hours

ADMINISTRATION:
- On empty stomach
- Chewable, dispersible tablets available in 25 mg, 50 mg, 100 mg, 150 mg tablets; instruct patient to thoroughly chew, manually crush, or disperse in at least 1 oz of water prior to swallowing. Tablets dissolve with stirring
- Buffered powder for oral solution available as a single dose foil packet in 100 mg, 167 mg and 250 mg packets. Instruct patient to carefully pour packet contents into 4 oz. of drinking water, NOT juice or acidic fluids, stir until dissolved, and to drink immediately
- Pediatric powder for oral solution is mixed by the pharmacist with purified water, USP, to an initial solution of 20 mg/mL, then further diluted with an antacid to a final concentration of 10 mg/mL

DRUG INTERACTIONS:
- Antacids: increases bioavailability of ddI
- Ciprofoxacin, other quinolone antibiotics, tetracycline: decreases antibiotic absorption; administer antibiotics 2 hours before ddI
- Dapsone: decreases absorption of dapsone; administer 2 hours apart
- Ketoconazole: decreased absorption of ketoconazole; administer 2 hours apart
- IV pentamidine: increased risk of pancreatitis; hold ddI during period of treatment with IV pentamidine

ADVERSE EFFECTS:
- Pancreatitis (incidence 9%, may be fatal)
- Peripheral neuropathy (34%)
- Hyperuricemia (50% of patients with preexisting hyperuricemia)
- Diarrhea (34%)
- Retinal depigmentation and visual changes in children (rare)
- Hepatic failure, cardiomyopathy (rare)
- Rash, pruritis

SPECIAL NURSING CONSIDERATIONS:
- in terms of increasing CD_4 counts, delaying AIDS diagnosis, and decreasing number of opportunistic infections
  —Zidovudine (AZT) superior to didanosine (ddI) in previously untreated patients
  —ddI superior to AZT in patients treated with AZT for > 4 months (ACTG 116, 117)
- Treatment with ddI after a prolonged course of AZT may make the HIV virus susceptible to AZT again
- Drug should be discontinued if patient developes signs/symptoms of pancreatitis
- Drug continuation should be evaluated if patient developes peripheral neuropathy; assess for signs/symptoms of peripheral neuropathy at each visit
- All children should receive dilated retinal exams every 6 months and whenever a change in vision occurs to identify retinal depigmentation

PATIENT EDUCATION:
- Drug not a cure for HIV but prevents viral replication
- Report all changes in condition (physical and mental)
- Peripheral neuropathy and pancreatitis are uncommon and are more likely to occur in individuals with a history of either
- Assess for and report signs/symptoms of neuropathy: numbness and burning, dysesthesia of distal extremities, and, if drug is continued, sharp, shooting pains or severe continuous burning
- Assess for and report signs/symptoms of pancreatitis: nausea, vomiting, abdominal pain

Diphenhydramine Hydrochloride

BRAND NAME:
- Benadryl

ACTION:
- Antihistamine, with sedative properties

INDICATIONS:
- Allergic disorders; used to reverse dystonic reactions to phenothiazine antiemetic (dopamine antagonist) agents, and to promote sleep

CONTRAINDICATIONS:
- Hypersensitivity to drug or other H_1-receptor antagonists
- Acute asthma attack
- Lower respiratory tract disease

DOSAGE:
- *Adult:*
  —Oral: 25–50 mg q 4 hours
  —IM: 25–50 mg q 4 hours
  —IV: 50 mg prior to chemotherapy or 25 mg q 4 hours X 4, beginning prior to antiemetic

ADMINISTRATION:
- Oral, with or without food, IM or IV

DRUG INTERACTIONS:
- CNS depressants: increase sedation; monitor patient closely

ADVERSE EFFECTS:
- Sedation, drowsines, dizziness, confusion
- Blurred vision/diplopia
- Dry mouth
- Urinary retention
- Rash, photosensitivity (uncommon)

SPECIAL NURSING CONSIDERATIONS:
- IV administration rapidly reverses extrapyramidal side effects

PATIENT EDUCATION:
- Avoid driving vehicle (e.g., car) when feel drowsy
- Avoid prolonged sun exposure

Diphenoxylate Hydrochloride and Atropine

BRAND NAMES:
- Lofene, Lomenate, Lomotil, Lonox

ACTION:
- Synthetic opiate; slows peristalsis, so excess water is absorbed from feces

INDICATIONS:
- Temporary relief from diarrhea

CONTRAINDICATIONS:
- Known hypersensitivity
- Obstructive jaundice
- Pseudomembranous colitis
- Diarrhea due to enterotoxin-producing bacteria
- Use with extreme caution in patients with hepatic coma, acute ulcerative colitis

DOSAGE:
- *Adults:* 5 mg PO qid until symptoms controlled, then titrated to individual's needs, often one-quarter of initial dosage

- Children (2–12 years): 0.3–0.4 mg/kg daily in 4 divided doses
- Decrease dose when diarrhea controlled

ADMINISTRATION:
- Oral: children should be given oral solution
- Available in tablets containing 2.5 mg diphenoxylate HCl and atropine 0.025 mg

DRUG INTERACTIONS:
- CNS depressants, alcohol: increases CNS depression; AVOID concurrent use or use cautiously
- MAO Inhibitiors: hypertensive crisis; AVOID concurrent use, or use cautiously

ADVERSE EFFECTS:
- Psychologic dependency when used in high doses (40–60 mg)
- Nausea, diarrhea, anorexia, mouth dryness
- Sedation, lethargy, restlessness
- Rash, pruritis, angioedema

SPECIAL NURSING CONSIDERATIONS:
- If no response in 48 hours, drug not effective
- Do not exceed recommended dosage, especially in children, as respiratory depression, coma, brain damage has occurred

PATIENT EDUCATION:
- Report rash, swelling immediately
- Do not exceed recommended dosage

Drug Profiles

- Report if diarrhea continues after 48 hours as alternative drug needs to be used
- Increase oral fluids to 3 L/day

Doxorubicin

BRAND NAME:
- Adriamycin

ACTION:
- Antineoplastic antibiotic; binds to DNA base pairs, and inhibits DNA and RNA synthesis

INDICATIONS:
- Breast cancer, multiple myeloma
- Used in treatment of Kaposi's sarcoma

CONTRAINDICATIONS:
- Known hypersensitivity
- Neutropenia, thrombocytopenia

DOSAGE:
- HIV: Kaposi's sarcoma:
  —Doxorubicin 10–20 mg/m^2 IV in combination with Bleomycin and Vincristine (ABV) q 2 weeks

ADMINISTRATION:
- Drug is a potent VESICANT
- Give slow IVP via freely running IV with excellent blood return confirmed throughout according to institutional guidelines

- Drug should be administered only by a NURSE SKILLED IN ADMINISTRATION OF CHEMO-THERAPY TREATMENT
- USE SAFE CHEMOTHERAPY HANDLING GUIDELINES; see Appendix I

DRUG INTERACTIONS:
- Heparin, 5 fluorouracil: forms precipitate; flush IV tubing with 0.9% NS between drugs
- Barbiturates: increases plasma clearance of doxorubicin
- Cyclophosphamide (high doses): increased risk of cardiotoxicity

ADVERSE EFFECTS:
- Pink urine X 48 hours
- Ulceration, pain, tissue necrosis if drug extravasates
- Nausea, vomiting
- Mucositis, alopecia
- Leukopenia, thrombocytopenia (nadir 10–14 days) especially with normal doses
- Cardiomyopathy (cumulative dose 550 mg/m^2)

SPECIAL NURSING CONSIDERATIONS:
- Doses are reduced in HIV-related patients because patients are taking other drugs, such as antiretroviral agent zidovudine, which may decrease WBC

- Less toxicity in HIV patients since dose is reduced
- BE FAMILIAR WITH INSTITUTION'S POLICY AND PROCEDURE FOR IV ADMINISTRATION OF VESICANT CHEMOTHERAPY

PATIENT EDUCATION:
- Report any pain, stinging, burning during drug administration immediately
- Oral hygiene after meals and at bedtime; report oral discomfort, ulcers
- Urine will be pink X 48 hours
- Report fever, bleeding, immediately

Doxycycline Hydrochloride

BRAND NAMES:
- Vibramycin, Doxy-Caps, Doryx

ACTION:
- Tetracycline-like antibiotic

INDICATIONS:
- Infections caused by sensitive gram-negative and gram-positive organisms
- Chlamydial and mycoplasmal infections
- Gonorrhea in individuals allergic to penicillin, cephalosporins, or probenecid
- Syphilis
- Rickettsial infections

CONTRAINDICATIONS:
- Known hypersensitivity to drug or tetracyclines
- Pregnancy, nursing mothers

DOSAGE:
- Oral:
  —*Adults, children* (> 8 years weighing > 45 kg): 100 mg q 12 hours day 1, then 100 mg q d in 1 or 2 divided doses
  —Chlamydia: 100 mg bid X 7 days
  —Gonorrhea/Syphilis: 300 mg/day in divided doses X 10 days
- IV:
  —200 mg IV day 1, then 100–200 mg q d

ADMINISTRATION:
- Oral, give with full glass of fluid
- Parenteral, administer over at least 60 minutes (100 mg); resume oral administration as soon as possible

DRUG INTERACTIONS:
- Coumadin: increases prothrombin time (PT); decrease coumadin dose
- Penicillin: decreases activity of penicillin; avoid concurrent use
- Antacids, iron-containing preparations: interfere with drug absorbtion; do not give concurrently

ADVERSE EFFECTS:
* Rash, photosensitivity (exaggerated sunburn)
* *Uncommon:*
  —Diarrhea, anorexia, nausea, vomiting
  —Superinfection by candida in anogenital region
  —Esophagitis, ulceration when drug taken at bedtime
  —Neutropenia, thrombocytopenia

SPECIAL NURSING CONSIDERATIONS:
* Drug can be given in patients with renal insufficiency safely

PATIENT EDUCATION:
* Take drug with large glass of water
* Do not take drug at bedtime
* Avoid exposure to direct sunlight, use sunblock, protective clothing
* Stop drug and report rash if this develops
* Do not take antacids or iron-containing vitamins

Econazole Nitrate 1% Cream

BRAND NAME:
* Spectazole (with benzoic acid)

ACTION:
* Antifungal agent with some antibacterial activity; interferes with micro-organism cell membrane integrity

INDICATIONS:
- Tinea pedis, tinea cruris, tinea corporis, cutaneous candidiasis, tinea versicolor

CONTRAINDICATIONS:
- Known hypersensitivity
- Use with caution in pregnancy or nursing mothers only if benefit exceeds risk

DOSAGE:
- Apply amount sufficient to cover affected area q d for tinea infections; apply bid for cutaneous candidiasis
- Duration: cutaneous candida, tinea cruris and corporis X 2 weeks; tinea pedis X 1 month

ADMINISTRATION:
- EXTERNAL USE ONLY
- AVOID contact with eyes, other mucous membranes including vagina

DRUG INTERACTIONS:
- Hydrocortisone, triamcinolone acetonide: inhibit antifungal activity of cream; avoid concurrent use

ADVERSE EFFECTS:
- *Uncommon* (3% of patients) :
  —Burning
  —Erythema
  —Itching
  —Stinging

SPECIAL NURSING CONSIDERATIONS:
- Clinical improvement, symptom relief expected within 1–2 weeks

PATIENT EDUCATION:
- Self-application of cream

Ethambutol Hydrochloride

BRAND NAME:
- Myambutol

ACTION:
- Antituberculosis agent; inhibits synthesis of cellular metabolites during cell division, resulting in cell death

INDICATIONS:
- Pulmonary tuberculosis, in combination with at least one other agent

CONTRAINDICATIONS:
- Known hypersensitivity
- Optic neuritis
- Children < 13 years old
- Use with caution in pregnancy

DOSAGE:
- *Adult initial treatment:* 15 mg/kg; 500 mg–1 gm q d in single dose
  —Retreatment: 25 mg/kg q d in single dose X 60 days, then 15 mg/kg

—when given with other drugs 2 X/week
instead of daily, dose is 50 mg/kg 2 X/week
* *Children, ages 6–13:* (not recommended by
manufacturer): 10–15 mg/kg with monthly
ophtalmologic testing
* Modify dose if renal impairment

ADMINISTRATION:
* Oral, available as 100 mg, 400 mg tablets
* Can take with food

DRUG INTERACTIONS:
* None known

ADVERSE EFFECTS:
* Dizziness
* Reversible optic neuritis in prolonged therapy
* Fever
* Dermatitis, pruritis
* Confusion, disorientation
* Headache
* Anaphylaxis (rare)
* Malaise, myalgia

SPECIAL NURSING CONSIDERATIONS:
* Duration of therapy usually 6–9 months
* Assess visual acuity baseline and periodically
during treatment (monthly if dose > 15 mg/kg)
using Snellen eye chart; discontine drug if
demonstrable worsening of visual acuity

- After drug discontinued, visual acuity usually returns to baseline over weeks to months. Drug has been reinstituted without loss of visual acuity
- Monitor serum BUN, creatinine, liver function tests, and CBC baseline and periodically during long-term therapy

PATIENT EDUCATION:
- Eye exams q month on dose of 25 mg/kg/day
- Report immediately any changes in visual acuity, blurred vision
- Need for compliance with long-term therapy

Ethionamide

BRAND NAME:
- Trecator–SC

ACTION:
- Antimycobacterial agent; inhibits peptide synthesis, preventing cell division

INDICATIONS:
- Active tuberculosis unresponsive to first-line agents (e.g., isoniazid streptomycin, aminosalicylic acid); given in combination with other agents

CONTRAINDICATIONS:
- Known hypersensitivity (severe)
- Hepatic insufficiency/failure
- Pregnancy
- Nursing mothers unless benefit > risk

DOSAGE:
- *Adult:* 0.5 gm–1.0 gm/day in 1–3 equally divided doses
- Administer with pyridoxine HCL

ADMINISTRATION:
- Oral; can give in divided doses or at bedtime as a single dose
- Available in 250 mg tablets

DRUG INTERACTIONS:
- Cycloserine, isoniazid: possible increase CNS toxicity; use together with caution and monitor closely

ADVERSE EFFECTS:
- Nausea, vomiting, diarrhea, abdominal pain, anorexia
- Depression, restlessness, dizziness, headache
- Rare peripheral neuritis, paresthesia, seizures, optic neuritis, blurred vision—prevent with concurrent administration of pyridoxine HCl
- Hepatotoxicity, especially in patients with diabetes mellitus
- Hypersensitivity (rash, photosensitivity, thrombocytopenia, purpura)

SPECIAL NURSING CONSIDERATIONS:
- GI side effects may be ameliorated by decreasing dose, giving as single dose at bedtime, or giving in divided doses with meals
- Use antiemetics to prevent nausea/vomiting; if ineffective, drug may need to be discontinued
- Monitor liver function tests baseline and q 2–4 weeks during therapy

PATIENT EDUCATION:
- Report nausea, vomiting; change drug administration schedule and/or take antinausea medicines as ordered
- Report changes in mood, dizziness
- Importance of taking pyridoxine HCl with meds as ordered
- Report any changes in condition

Epoetin alfa

BRAND NAME:
- Procrit

ACTION:
- Recombinant glycoprotein (erythropoietin) that stimulates red blood cell production in the bone marrow

INDICATIONS:
- Anemia in AZT (zidovudine)-treated HIV patients

- Anemia in chronic renal failure patients
- Anemia in patients receiving myelosuppressive chemotherapy

CONTRAINDICATIONS:
- Hypersensitivity to albumin
- Uncontrolled hypertension
- Patients with endogenous erythropoietin level > 500 mμ/mL

DOSAGE:
- 100 μ/kg SC or IV 3 X/week X 8 weeks
- If hematocrit does not increase, increase dose by 50–100 μ/kg 3X/week to max 300 μ/kg 3 X/week
- Interrupt therapy if hematocrit ≥ 40%, resume again at 75% of dose when hematocrit ≤ 36%

ADMINISTRATION:
- Subcutaneous injection or IV. DO NOT shake vial as it may denature glycoprotein
- Available in single use vials containing 2000, 3000, 4000, or 10,000 units (U)

DRUG INTERACTIONS:
- None reported

ADVERSE EFFECTS:
- Pyrexia, fatigue, headache (may be due to HIV disease)
- Polycythemia if target and hematocrit of 40 exceeded

Drug Profiles

SPECIAL NURSING CONSIDERATIONS:
- Best effect in patients receiving AZT ≤ 4200 mg/ week
- Assess patient's ability to administer SC injections
- Involve home care nurses as needed

PATIENT EDUCATION:
- Drug preparation, subcutaneous injection technique, and disposal of used equipment

Erythromycin base

BRAND NAMES:
- E-mycin, Robimycin, Robitabs

ACTION:
- Antibiotic, bacteriostatic through inhibition of protein synthesis

INDICATIONS:
- Streptococcal infections of respiratory tract, skin, and soft tissues by sensitive organisms
- Syphilis in patients unable to take penicillin or tetracycline

CONTRAINDICATIONS:
- Known hypersensitivity
- Use with caution in patients with hepatic dysfunction or impaired biliary function, pregnant women, nursing mothers

DOSAGE:
- *Adult:* 250 mg q 6 hours or 333 mg q 8 hours
- *Children:* 30–50 mg/kg daily in 4 divided doses
- In severe infections total dose may be 4 gm for adults, 60–100 mg/kg/day for children

ADMINISTRATION:
- Oral, give on empty stomach
- Available in enteric coated, 250 mg, 333 mg, and 500 mg tabs

DRUG INTERACTIONS:
- Carbamazepine: increase carbamazepine toxicity; monitor for ataxia, dizziness, vomiting and adjust dose
- Cyclosporine: increase cyclosporine levels; monitor for neurotoxicity
- Theophylline (high dose): increased theophylline levels; monitor closely
- Warfarin: may increase prothrombin time (PT); monitor PT closely

ADVERSE EFFECTS:
- Nausea, vomiting, diarrhea, abdominal pain, cramping
- Rash, fever, urticaria

SPECIAL NURSING CONSIDERATIONS:
* Assess for superinfection by nonsusceptible microorganisms (e.g., fungi)

PATIENT EDUCATION:
* Report rash
* Take drug 1 hour before or 2 hours after meals

Etoposide (VP-16)

BRAND NAME:
* Vepesid

ACTION:
* Antineoplastic agent; inhibits DNA synthesis, preventing mitosis, and causing cell death

INDICATIONS:
* Refractory testicular cancer; small cell lung cancer
* May be used in the treatment of Kaposi's sarcoma (not indicated by Food and Drug Administration)

CONTRAINDICATIONS:
* Known hypersensitivity
* Cytopenias (granulocytopenia, thrombocytopenia)
* Pregnancy

DOSAGE:

- Kapsoi's sarcoma: 50–100 mg/m^2 IV q d X 3, every 3–4 weeks or 50 mg PO q d X 14–21 days, depending on neutrophil count

ADMINISTRATION:

- Premedicate with antiemetic agent
- IV: dilute to concentration of 0.2 mg/mL or 0.4 mg/mL, and administer over 30–60 minutes or longer. Monitor for hypotension (slow drug infusion rate if this occurs) and bronchospasm (stop drug and discontinue if this occurs)
- Oral: administer oral antiemetic 1 hour before oral dose
- Should only be administered by NURSE SKILLED IN CHEMOTHERAPY ADMINISTRATION
- USE CHEMOTHERAPY HANDLING PRECAUTIONS

DRUG INTERACTIONS:

- Other myelosuppressive drugs: increased toxicity; avoid concurrent use or use neutrophil accelerating agent, e.g., G-CSF (filgastrim)

ADVERSE EFFECTS:

- Alopecia (reversible)
- Nausea, vomiting (mild)
- Neutropenia, thrombocytopenia; nadir 7–14 days
- Peripheral neuropathy
- Anaphylaxis (rare)

SPECIAL NURSING CONSIDERATIONS:
- Response in Kaposi's sarcoma 75%
- Radiation recall may occur if combined therapies given
- USE SAFE HANDLING PRECAUTIONS (SEE APPENDIX I)
- Nausea/vomiting may be increased with oral dosage of drug

PATIENT EDUCATION:
- Alopecia reversible, hair will grow back
- Assess for signs/symptoms infection, bleeding, and report immediately
- Take antinausea pill prior to oral dose

Filgrastim (G-CSF)

BRAND NAME:
- Neupogen

ACTION:
- Recombinant cytokine; stimulates production and maturation of neutrophil precursors in the bone marrow

INDICATIONS:
- Acceleration of neutrophil recovery after cancer chemotherapy to prevent febrile neutropenia

CONTRAINDICATIONS:
- Hypersensitivity to *E. coli* derived protein

DOSAGE:
- 5 µg/kg/day SC or IV, beginning at least 24 hours postchemotherapy, continuing up to 2 weeks or until ANC $\geq$ 10,000/mm^3

ADMINISTRATION:
- Subcutaneous injection
- Can be given IV but may need to be mixed with albumin to prevent adsorption to IV tubing
- DO NOT SHAKE VIAL

DRUG INTERACTIONS:
- None significant

ADVERSE EFFECTS:
- Transient skeletal bone pain
- Rash (uncommon)

SPECIAL NURSING CONSIDERATIONS:
- Bone pain due to expansion of bone marrow cells' response to G-CSF
- Monitor WBC, absolute neutrophil count (ANC) 2 X/week during therapy. Dose should be discontinued when ANC $\geq$ 10,000/mm^3
- Contact Amgen representative for patient teaching video, booklets in English and Spanish (subcutaneous injection)

PATIENT EDUCATION:
- Take nonsteroidal anti-inflammatory drug as ordered to relieve bone pain

- Drug preparation, subcutaneous injection technique, and disposal of used equipment
- Report rash

Fluconazole

BRAND NAME:
- Diflucan

ACTION:
- Antifungal agent; inhibits fungal enzyme system, causing fungal death

INDICATIONS:
- Oropharyngeal and esophageal candidiasis
- Cryptococcal meningitis

CONTRAINDICATIONS:
- Known hypersensitivity to drug

DOSAGE:
- Candidiasis: 200 mg PO day 1, then 100 mg q d 2 weeks (oropharyngeal); X 3 weeks for esophageal, then 2 weeks after symptoms resolve; may be titrated up to 400 mg PO based on patient's response
- Systemic candidiasis: 400 mg day 1, then 200 mg q d X 4 or more weeks, then X 2 weeks after symptoms resolve
- Cryptococcal infections: initial: 400 mg day 1, then 200–400 mg q d X 10–12 weeks after

cerebrospinal fluid (CSF) cultures are negative for cryptococcus; maintenance: 200 mg q d indefinitely
- Dose reduce if renal impariment exists

ADMINISTRATION:
- Oral is preferred route; without regard to food intake
- Available in 50 mg, 100 mg, and 200 mg tablets
- IV dose should be infused over 1 hour

DRUG INTERACTIONS:
- Coumadin: $\uparrow$ prothrombin time (PT); monitor PT closely and adjust coumadin dose as needed
- Cyclosporine: $\uparrow$ serum levels; monitor for cyclosporin toxicity
- Phenytoin: $\uparrow$ serum levels; monitor for phenytoin toxicity and $\downarrow$ dose
- Rifampin: $\uparrow$ fluconazole serum levels; $\uparrow$ fluconazole dose when given together
- Sulfonylureas: $\uparrow$ hypoglycemia; monitor serum glucose levels
- Rifampin, isoniazid: $\uparrow$ risk of hepatotoxicity; monitor liver function tests

ADVERSE EFFECTS:
- Adverse effects more common in HIV-infected patients, occurring in approximately 20% of patients
- Nausea, vomiting, diarrhea, abdominal pain
- Rash, eosinophilia, pruritis

- Mild increase in liver function tests, often normalizing with continued therapy
- Rarely, anaphylaxis, liver dysfunction, exfoliative dermatitis

SPECIAL NURSING CONSIDERATIONS:
- Drug is generally well tolerated
- Monitor liver function tests (LFTs) baseline and periodically during therapy
- If abnormal LFTs occur, monitor patient closely for signs/symptoms of liver disease and discontinue drug
- If rash develops, monitor patient closely and discontinue drug if rash progresses
- Drug absorption is NOT affected by gastric pH as with ketoconazole

PATIENT EDUCATION:
- Take drug without regard to meals
- Report rash immediately
- Report nausea, vomiting, abdominal pain, yellowing of skin or sclerae immediately

Flucytosine

BRAND NAME:
- Ancobon

ACTION:
- Nonantibiotic antifungal agent; is converted to fluorouracil in fungal cells and interferes with RNA and DNA synthesis

INDICATIONS:
- Serious infections caused by *Candida* or *Cryptococcus*; usually alternative to first-line therapies

CONTRAINDICATIONS:
- Known hypersensitivity
- Use with extreme caution when renal impairment or bone marrow suppression exists

DOSAGE:
- 50–150 mg/kg q d in 4 equally divided doses q 6 hours

ADMINISTRATION:
- Oral, give capsules over 15 minute period
- Available in 250 mg capsules

DRUG INTERACTIONS:
- Cytosine arabinoside: inhibits flucytosine
- Amphotericin B: possible synergism

ADVERSE EFFECTS:
- *Common:*
  —Nausea, vomiting, diarrhea, abdominal discomfort, ulcerative colitis
- *Occasional:*
  —Bone marrow suppression with leukopenia, thrombocytopenia
  —Hepatitis (dose-related)
  —Rash

—Confusion
—Hypokalemia
* *Rare:*
  —Anaphylaxis
  —Cardiac, respiratory arrest

SPECIAL NURSING CONSIDERATIONS:
* Monitor serum potassium, CBC, renal and hepatic function baseline and periodically during treatment
* Optimal serum level 25–120 µg/mL
* Risk of bone marrow suppression increases with prolonged, high serum levels of ≥ 100 µg/ mL, renal impairment, or concurrent administration with Amphoterin B
* Safety in children has not been established, but for children weighing < 50 kg, doses of 1.5–4.5 gm/m^2 q d have been used

PATIENT EDUCATION:
* Need for frequent blood monitoring
* Report signs/symptoms of infection, bleeding immediately
* Take antiemetic to reduce nausea/vomiting as ordered; report severe or persistent symptoms
* Take capsules over 15 minute periods

Fluoxetine Hydrochloride

BRAND NAME:
- Prozac

ACTION:
- Antidepressant (selectively inhibits reuptake of serotonin)

INDICATIONS:
- Major depression
- Obsessive compulsive disorder
- Bipolar disorder
- Panic attacks
- Obesity
- Myoclonus
- Eating disorders

CONTRAINDICATIONS:
- Use with caution in patients with:
  —Hepatic dysfunction
  —Renal dysfunction; may need to dose reduce—see package insert
  —patients with recent MI
- Hypersensitivity

DOSAGE:
- *Adult:* 20 mg q d maintenance (may start with 5mg q d or 20 mg q 2–3 days)
- May be titrated up according to response

ADMINISTRATION:
- Orally without regard to meals

DRUG INTERACTIONS:
- Monamine oxidase inhibitors: AVOID concurrent use
- Tricyclic antidepressants: sedation, decreased energy: AVOID if possible
- Tryptophan: nausea, vomiting, disease, cramps: AVOID if possible
- Benzodiazepam: increases activity; avoid in elderly
- Buspirone: increases anxiety; use with caution
- Lithium: unclear: USE WITH CAUTION
- CNS agents: use together with caution

ADVERSE EFFECTS:
- Nausea
- Tremor
- Anxiety
- Dizziness
- Nervousness
- Sweating
- Insomnia
- Rash, pruritis
- Fatigue, asthenia
- Headaches

SPECIAL NURSING CONSIDERATIONS:
- Long elimination half-life of drug, so adverse side effects resolve slowly after drug withdrawn

- Closely supervise patients at high-risk for suicidal ideation/behavior—prescribe in smallest quantity possible
- Overdose may cause seizures
- Monitor blood sugar in diabetics and adjust hypoglycemic medicines
- 4 weeks to achieve maximum antidepression effect

PATIENT EDUCATION:
- Notify MD of all meds taken, including OTC
- Drug may impair activities requiring mental alertness
- Notify physician immediately if rash, hives develop

Foscarnet

BRAND NAME:
- Foscavir

ACTION:
- Antiviral, antiretroviral agent; inhibits viral DNA polymerase and reverse transcriptase, preventing replication of all *Herpes, Cytomegalovirus* (CMV), Epstein-Barr (EBV), and *Varicella zoster* (VSV) viruses

INDICATIONS:
- CMV retinitis in patients with AIDS

CONTRAINDICATIONS:
- Known hypersensitivity
- Pregnancy
- Nursing mothers

DOSAGE:
- Patients with normal renal function:
  —Induction: 60 mg /kg IV over 1 hour q 8 hours X 2–3 weeks
  —Maintenance: 90–120 mg/kg/day IV over 2 hours
  —Decrease dose in renal insufficiency

ADMINISTRATION:
- IV over 1–2 hours, using rate controller device
- Drug incompatible with D30W, lactated Ringer's solution

DRUG INTERACTIONS:
- Hypocalcemic agents: additive hypocalcemia; DO NOT USE TOGETHER
- Nephrotoxic drugs (gentamycin, amphotericin B): additive nephrotoxicity; AVOID CONCURRENT USE
- Pentamidine (IV): potentially fatal hypocalcemia; DO NOT USE TOGETHER
- Zidovudine: increase anemia; monitor patient closely, transfuse red blood cells as needed

ADVERSE EFFECTS:
- Renal insufficiency, renal failure
- Hypocalcemia, hypophosphatemia,

hyperphosphatemia, hypomagnesemia, hypokalemia
- Anemia
- Nausea, vomiting, diarrhea
- Neutropenia
- Rash
- Headache, paresthesia, neuropathy

SPECIAL NURSING CONSIDERATIONS:
- Monitor renal function (creatinine clearance) baseline, 2–3 X/week during *induction*; at least q 1–2 weeks during *maintenance* therapy (see Appendix III for formula)
- Dose reduce if renal insufficiency exists according to manufacturer's recommendations
- Monitor electrolytes, calcium, magnesium, phosphorus baseline 2–3 X/week during *induction,* and 1–2 X/week during *maintenance* treatment
- Monitor hemoglobin, hematocrit baseline and during treatment. Transfuse red blood cells as ordered
- Assess patient's self-care ability and need for home supports
- Administer antiemetics as ordered
- Monitor WBC, ANC and assess for signs/ symptoms of infection
- Useful in treating CMV resistant to ganciclovir

PATIENT EDUCATION:
- Report perioral tingling, numbness, paresthesia during or after infusion

- Report fatigue, activity intolerance
- Report signs/symptoms of infection

Ganciclovir

BRAND NAME:
- Cytovene

ACTION:
- Antiviral agent; prevents viral replication of *Cytomegalovirus* (CMV)

INDICATIONS:
- CMV retinitis
- CMV prophylaxis in patients receiving organ transplantation

CONTRAINDICATIONS:
- Known hypersensitivity to drug or acyclovir
- Pregnancy, nursing mothers
- Use with caution, if at all in patients with pre-existing cytopenias, or if receiving bone marrow suppressive agents
- Use with extreme caution in children

DOSAGE:
- *Adults, children > 3 months of age:*
  —CMV retinitis: treatment: 5.0 mg/kg IV q 12 hours X 14–21 days, then suppression therapy; post-therapy: 6.0 mg/kg IV q day x 5 days/week indefinitely

—Dose reduce if renal impairment exists (urine creatinine clearance < 80 mL/min)

ADMINISTRATION:
- Administer only if absolute neutrophil count (ANC) > 500/mm^3, and platelets are >25,000/mm^3
- Infuse IV over 1 hour, with ADEQUATE hydration and urinary output established
- Avoid extravasation
- USE SAFE CHEMOTHERAPY HANDLING TECHNIQUES (see Appendix I)

DRUG INTERACTIONS:
- Corticosteroids, cyclosprine: increases bone marrow depression; dose reduce or hold immunosuppressant drugs
- Cytotoxic chemotherapy: additive bone marrow depression, toxicity to gonads, GI mucosa; avoid concurrent use
- Other cytotoxic drugs (dapsone, pentamidine, flucytosine, amphotericin B, trimethoprim-sulfamethoxazole): increases toxicity; use cautiously and monitor patient closely
- Foscarnet: synergism
- Imipenem/cilastin: increases neurotoxicity with seizures; AVOID concurrent use
- Interferon: potent synergism against herpes virus, varicella-zoster virus
- Probenecid: may increase ganciclovir levels; monitor closely and decreases ganciclovir dose as needed

- Zidovudine: increases hematologic toxicity (neutropenia, anemia); avoid concurrent use, consider didanosine, and/or use granulocyte-macrophage colony stimulating factor to increase absolute neutrophil count (ANC)

ADVERSE EFFECTS:
- Neutropenia (25–50% of patients)
- Thrombocytopenia (20%)
- Retinal detachment (30%)
- Phlebitis
- Headache, confusion
- Increases liver function tests
- Rash
- Rarely, seizure, coma

SPECIAL NURSING CONSIDERATIONS:
- Drug is carcinogenic and mutagenic; USE SAFE HANDLING PRECAUTIONS (see Appendix I)
- Monitor absolute neutrophil count (see Appendix III for calculation) and platelet count, baseline and during therapy. Manufacturer recommends assessment of neutrophil and platelet counts every two days when dosing is bid, then at least weekly; monitoring should be daily if patient is neutropenic prior to therapy or if the patient has a prior history of leukopenia following ganciclovir or other similar drug therapy.

- Monitor BUN, serum creatinine, urine creatinine clearance weekly during therapy; reduce drug dose if renal dysfunction occurs
- Consider central line for ongoing drug therapy since vein irritation occurs
- Most HIV-infected patients develop progressive retinal necrosis within 1 month if initial treatment is not followed by lifetime suppressive therapy
- Patient should see an ophthalmologist at least q 6 weeks during therapy

PATIENT EDUCATION:
- Drug does not cure virus, and viral recurrence or progression
  can occur despite therapy
- Report any worsening of vision
- Report signs/symptoms of infection, bleeding immediately

Griseofulvin

BRAND NAMES:
- Grisactin, Grifulvin, Fulvicin, Gris-PEG

ACTION:
- Antifungal agent; destroys fungal mitotic spindle, causing metaphase arrest and cell death

INDICATIONS:

* Tinea (ringworm) infections of skin, hair, nails (tinea corporis, pedis, cruris, barbae, capitis, unguium)

CONTRAINDICATIONS:

* Porphyria
* Pregnant women
* Hepatocellular failure
* Nursing mothers
* Known hypersensitivity

DOSAGE:

* *Adult:*
   —Tinea corporis cruris, capitus: (ultramicro size) is 330–375 mg/day; (microsize) is 500 mg/day X 2–8 weeks
   —Tinea pedia and unguium (ultra micro size): 660–750 mg/day; (microsize) is 1 gm/day X 4–6 months
* Consult package insert for manufacturer's recommendations

ADMINISTRATION:

* Oral; single dose or in 2–4 divided doses

DRUG INTERACTIONS:

* Alcohol: potentiates alcohol effect (tachycardia, flushing, inebriation); avoid concurrent use
* Phenobarbital: decreases griseofulvin serum level; give griseofulvin in 3 divided doses and monitor serum level

- Warfarin: decreases prothrombin time; monitor PT closely, and modify warfarin dose
- Oral contraceptives: increases breakthrough bleeding, decreases contraceptive efficacy; use backup contraception

ADVERSE EFFECTS:
- Headache, may disappear with continued therapy
- Fatigue, dizziness, insomia
- Urticaria, rashes, photosensitivity
- *Rare:*
  —Paresthesias of hands and feet
  —Nausea, vomiting, diarrhea
  —Oral thrush (*Candida* overgrowth)
  —Renal, hepatic dysfunction
  —Granulocytopenia

SPECIAL NURSING CONSIDERATIONS:
- Drug is mutagenic and carcinogenic
- Not effective in treatment of tinea versicolor, candidiasis
- Second-line agent, used for resistant infections after trials with other topical antifungal agents
- Treatment depends on time needed for sloughing of infected keratinized sites. Soles, palms of hands, and nails require prolonged treatment
- Monitor renal, liver function studies and CBC baseline and periodically during treatment

PATIENT EDUCATION:
- Avoid exposure to strong sunlight
- Report any drug rash, numbness of hands or feet
- Use backup contraceptive (women taking contraceptives)

Haloperidol

BRAND NAME:
- Haldol

ACTION:
- Tranquilizer; depresses cerebral cortex, hypothalamus, limbic system; also acts as mild antiemetic by blocking dopamine receptors in chemotherapy receptor trigger zone (CTZ)

INDICATIONS:
- Management of psychotic disorders

CONTRAINDICATIONS:
- Severe toxic CNS depression or coma
- Known hypersensitivity
- Parkinson's disease
- Blood dyscrasias, brain damage, drug/alcohol withdrawal

DOSAGE:
- *Adult:* psychosis: 0.5–2 mg bid or tid; increase to 3–5 mg bid-tid for severe symptoms
- Antiemetic: 3–5 mg PO q 2 hours X 3–4 doses, beginning 30 minutes before chemotherapy

ADMINISTRATION:
- Oral: available as 0.5, 1, 2, 5, 10, 20 mg tabs
- IM: injectable available in 5 mg/mL ampules

DRUG INTERACTIONS:
- Epinephrine: reversal of vasopressor effects; avoid concurrent use
- CNS depressants: increases sedation; monitor closely

ADVERSE EFFECTS:
- Tardive dyskinesia (with long-term use)
- Orthostatic hypotension
- *Rare:*
  —Laryngospasm
  —Tachycardia, EKG changes

SPECIAL NURSING CONSIDERATIONS:
- As entiemetic, equivalent to tetrahydrocannabinol and superior to phenothiazines
- Assess for tardive dyskinesia with long-term use (involuntary movements, sedation, extrapyrimidal symptoms)
- If orthostatic hypotension occurs and patient is symptomatic, use metaraminol or norepinephrine to increase BP not epinephrine

PATIENT EDUCATION:
- Report sedation, involuntary movements, restlessness
- Change positions slowly

Hydromorphone Hydrochloride

BRAND NAME:
- Dilaudid

ACTION:
- Narcotic analgesic

INDICATIONS:
- Relief of moderate to severe pain

CONTRAINDICATIONS:
- Known hypersensitivity
- Intracranial tumors causing increased intracranial pressure
- Depressed pulmonary states

DOSAGE:
- Range:
  —Moderate pain: 1–6 mg PO q 4–6 hours; 2–4

mg IM; SC q 4–6 hours; 3 mg rectal suppository
q 6 hours
—Severe pain: 4+ mg PO/IM/SC q 4 hours

ADMINISTRATION:
- Use with caution in opiate-naive patients
- Titrate to relieve pain
- Oral form available in 2, 3, and 4 mg tablets

DRUG INTERACTIONS:
- Alcohol, CNS depressants: increases CNS
  depression; use with caution or AVOID if
  possible
- Acetaminophen, aspirin: increases additive
  analgesia; use to advantage
- Narcan: antagonism; use to reverse respiratory
  depression

ADVERSE EFFECTS:
- Drowsiness, sedation, mood changes
- Constipation
- Nausea, vomiting
- Orthostatic hypotension
- Bladder spasm
- Psychological dependence
- Impotence, decreased libido
- Rarely, respiratory depression

SPECIAL NURSING CONSIDERATIONS:
- Parenteral dose is one-quarter oral dose for
  equianalgesic effect

- Give dose necessary to relieve pain, but need to give the smallest effective dose to prevent development of tolerance, physical dependence
- Ensure patient is placed on bowel regime

PATIENT EDUCATION:
- Avoid alcohol
- Importance of bowel regime to move bowels at least every other day
- Increase oral fluids to 3L/day, foods high in fiber, exercise as tolerated
- Report unrelieved pain

Ibuprofen

BRAND NAMES:
- Advil, Ibuprin, Medipren, Motrin, Nuprin, Rufen

ACTION:
- Nonsteroidal inflammatory agent (NSAID); analgesic, anti-inflammatory, antipyretic activity probably due to prostaglandin inhibition

INDICATIONS:
- Relief of minor pain, inflammation, and fever

CONTRAINDICATIONS:
- Known hypersensitivity
- Aspirin-hypersensitivity reaction (cross-reactivity)
- Gastric or duodenal ulcers
- Use cautiously, if at all, in renal impairment

DOSAGE:
- *Adult:* 200–800 mg q 4–8 hours or 3–4 X/day (max 3.2 gm/day)
- *Children:* (6 months–12 years): 5–10 mg/kg (max 40 mg/kg/day)

ADMINISTRATION:
- Oral: take with milk or food
- Available in 200, 300, 400, 600, 800 mg tablets and oral suspension 100 mg/5 mL

DRUG INTERACTIONS:
- Aspirin, other NSAID: increases risk of GI bleeding; avoid concurrent use
- Furosemide, thiazide diuretics: decreased diuretic effect
- Oral anticoagulants, thrombolytic agents: increased prothrombin time; monitor for bleeding, decrease dose; AVOID concurrent use if possible

ADVERSE EFFECTS:
- Dyspepsia, heartburn, nausea, vomiting, constipation
- Dizziness, headache, lightheadedness, fatigue
- Elevated liver function tests (15% patients)
- Rash
- Renal failure if preexisting renal dysfunction

SPECIAL NURSING CONSIDERATIONS:
- Factors increasing risk of bleeding: smoking, alcoholism

- Monitor baseline and periodic liver function tests, as well as hemoglobin/hematocrit if receiving prolonged course of drug
- Monitor patients with renal dysfunction very closely; baseline and periodic BUN/serum creatinine

PATIENT EDUCATION:
- Take with milk or food
- Increased risk of bleeding with smoking, alcohol ingestion
- Report bleeding, abdominal pain, jaundice, black stools immediately
- DO NOT TAKE with aspirin, other NSAIDs

Imipenem-Cilastatin

BRAND NAME:
- Primaxin

ACTION:
- Broad specrum beta-lactam antibiotic, active against most aerobic and anaerobic gram-positive and gram-negative organisms; useful against resistant strains

INDICATIONS:
- Serious infections of lower respiratory tract, urinary tract, abdomen, gynecologic tract, skin and bone

CONTRAINDICATIONS:

- Known hypersensitivity to imipenem-cilastatin, or severe hypersensitivity to penicillin
- IM: known hypersensitivity to lidocaine

DOSAGE:

- *Adults:*
  —IV: 250mg–1 gm q 6–8 hours to maximum 50 mg/kg or 4 gm/day, whichever is less
  —IM (if unable to give IV): 500–700 mg q 12 hours (max 1.5 gm/day)
- Dose reduce if renal impairment exists

ADMINISTRATION:

- IV mix: in 100 mL 5% dextrose injection or 0.9% sodium chloride IV over 60 minutes
- IM:
  —Reconstitute with lidocaine HCl 1% (without epinephrine) as recommended by manufacturer
  —Give deep IM into large muscle mass
  —DO NOT USE IM preparation for IV use

DRUG INTERACTIONS:

- Aminoglycosides: synergism
- Beta-lactam antibiotics (cephalosporins, extended spectrum penicillins): antagonism; do not use concurrently
- Ganciclovir: may decrease seizure threshold; do not use concurrently if possible
- Probenecid: increases antibiotic serum levels

ADVERSE EFFECTS:
- Rash, pruritis, urticaria
- Nausea, vomiting, diarrhea
- Fungal superinfection (e.g., vaginal moniliasis)
- Sterile abcess at IM injection site; phlebitis when given IV
- Rarely, pseudomembranous colitis, leukopenia, dizziness

SPECIAL NURSING CONSIDERATIONS:
- Usually used in combination with other antibiotics, such as an aminoglycoside
- Increased risk of allergic reaction if allergy to penicillin exists
- Assess for signs/symptoms of fungal overgrowth of mucous membranes

PATIENT EDUCATION:
- Increased risk for candidal infections of mucous membranes
- Self-assess for signs/symptoms
- Report rash

Interferon alfa (IFN alpha)

BRAND NAMES:
- Roferon-A, Intron A, Alferon N

ACTION:
- Recombinant cytokine with antiviral, antiproliferative, and immunomodulatory actions

INDICATIONS:
- Roferon-A: AIDS-related Kaposi's sarcoma (KS); hairy cell leukemia
- Intron A: AIDS-related KS, hairy cell leukemia, chronic non-A, non-B/C hepatitis, chronic hepatitis B (compensated)
- Alferon N: intralesional treatment of refractory or recurrent external condylomata acuminata

CONTRAINDICATIONS:
- Hypersensitivity to drug
- Anaphylactit sensitivity to mouse immuno-globulin

DOSAGE:
- AIDS-related Kaposi's sarcoma
  —Roferon-A (IFN-2a): 5–12 million IU (MIU) SC q d in combination with an antiretroviral agent
  —Intron A (IFN-2b): 5–10 MIU sc q d in combination with an antiretroviral agent
- Condylomata acuminata:
  —Alferon N: 0.05 mL (2.5 million IU) per wart 2 X/week X up to 8 weeks
  —Intron A: 0.1 mL (1 million IU from 10 MIU vial) per wart 3 X/week X 3 weeks

ADMINISTRATION:
- AIDS-related Kaposi's Sarcoma: subcutaneous injection or Intramuscular
  —Rofern-A : available in 3 MIU/vial or 18 MIU/ multidose vial

Drug Profiles   **157**

—Intron A : available in powder for injection (3-, 5-, 10-, 25-, 50-MIU vials)
- *Condylomata acuminata:*
  —Alferon N: injected into the wart base, using a 30-gauge needle (intralesional, external condylomata acuminata); available in vial containing 5 million IU/mL
  —Intron A: injected using 25–30 gauge needle into dermal core, 3 X/week X 3 weeks
- DO NOT SHAKE VIAL OR FREEZE

DRUG INTERACTIONS:
- Theophylline: increase serum levels; monitor closely and dose reduce
- Zidovudine: synergy but increased bone marrow toxicity; monitor patient labs closely
- CNS depressants: may increase CNS effects; monitor patient closely

ADVERSE EFFECTS:
- Flu-like syndrome (myalgias, fever, headache)
- Neutropenia, thrombocytopenia
- Anorexia, may be severe
- Mild nausea
- Diarrhea
- Dizziness, confusion, depression
- Dose-related increase in renal, hepatic function tests
- Rash, partial alopecia

SPECIAL NURSING CONSIDERATIONS:
- Monitor WBC, absolute neutrophil count (see Appendix III) and platelet count, as well as renal and hepatic function tests, baseline and periodically during treatment
- Warts (*Condylomata acuminata*) begin to disappear a few weeks after treatment begins, and continue to resolve after treatment completed; toxicity limited to flu-like syndrome
- Tolerance to nausea occurs after 1 week

PATIENT EDUCATION:
- Self-injection technique (KS)
- Assess for signs/symptoms of infection, bleeding; report this immediately
- Take acetaminophen or nonsteroidal anti-inflammatory drugs as ordered to enhance comfort
- Report any changes in mood or in general condition
- Report any rash

Iodoquinol

BRAND NAMES:
- Yodoxin, Diquinol, Yodoquinol

ACTION:
- Iodine containing luminal amebicide

INDICATIONS:
- Treatment of intestinal amebiasis
- Useful in treatment of *Entameoba histolytica, Blastocystis hominis, Dientamoeba fragilis*

CONTRAINDICATIONS:
- Hypersensitivity
- Patients with thyroid disease (use with caution)
- Hepatic or renal disease, preexisting optic neuropathy
- Pregnancy, nursing mothers

DOSAGE:
- *Adult:* 630–650 mg tid X 20 days (max 2 gm/day)
- If adult is also receiving other agents to treat hepatic abcess, use pedidose
- *Children:* 30–40 mg/kg or 1 gm/m^2 in 2–3 divided doses/day X 20 days (max 1.956 gm)

ADMINISTRATION:
- Orally, after meals; may be crushed and mixed with applesauce or chocolate syrup
- Do not repeat for 2–3 weeks
- Available in powder (Yodoxin) or tablets: Yodoxin (210 mg) or Diquinil (650 mg)

DRUG INTERACTIONS:
- None known

ADVERSE EFFECTS:
- Furunculosis
- Fever, headache
- Urticaria
- Anorexia
- Pruritis
- Nausea, vomiting, diarrhea
- Thyroid enlargement
- Abdominal cramps, gastritis
- Neurotoxicity (related to dose, duration of treatment)
- Optic neuritis, optic atrophy, peripheral neuropathy especially in children
- Weakness, dysesthesias
- Agitation, retrograde amnesia
- Subacute myelo-optic neuropathy = SMON— syndrome of muscle pain, weakness, optic atrophy, and ataxia (large doses for prolonged periods)

SPECIAL NURSING CONSIDERATIONS:
- May be used as drug of choice for asymptomatic cyst passers, or may be used following metronidazole for treatment of mild–moderate intestinal disease
- Should be used together with a tissue amebicide for the treatment of severe or acute forms of disease
- If rash occurs, notify MD but do not discontinue drug
- Drug may interfere with thyroid treatment tests X 6 months

Drug Profiles   **161**

PATIENT EDUCATION:
- Report rash, visual changes immediately
- Report itching, nausea, vomiting, diarrhea, any changes in condition

Isoniazid (INH)

BRAND NAMES:
- Laniazid; Tubizid; Hydrazid

ACTION:
- Antimycobacterial agent; interferes with cellular metabolism, resulting in loss of cell wall integrity

INDICATIONS:
- Tuberculosis (TB); must be combined with at least one other agent

CONTRAINDICATIONS:
- Known hypersensitivity, including drug-induced hepatitis, drug fever with chills, arthritis
- Use in pregnant women or nursing mothers only when benefit outweighs risk

DOSAGE:
- *Adults:* 5–10 mg/kg/day (maximum 300 mg/day); if given 2 X/week, dose is 15 mg/kg (up to 900 mg) 2 X/week
- *Children:* 10–20 mg/kg/day (maximum 300–500 mg/day; decrease dose if combined with rifampin

ADMINISTRATION:
- Oral; IM if oral route not feasible
- TB treatment duration: 6–9 months
- TB prophylaxis: 6–12 months

DRUG INTERACTIONS:
- Aluminum hydroxide gel: decreases INH absorption; give INH > 1 hour before antacid
- Cycloserine, ethionamide: increases neurotoxicity; monitor patient closely
- Carbamazepine: increases carbamazepine serum levels during initiation of INH therapy; monitor closely for carbamazepine toxicity (ataxia, headache, blurred vision, confusion) and modify dose
- Disulfiram: incoordination; avoid concurrent use
- Phenytoin: increases serum levels of phenytoin; monitor closely, decreasephenytoin dose

ADVERSE EFFECTS:
- Severe hepatitis (age-related risk, can be fatal)
- Mild hepatic dysfunction (mild, transient increases AST (SGOT), ALT (SGPT), bilirubin, during first 4–6 months, returning to normal on therapy
- Sensitivity reactions: fever, rash, lymphadenopathy, vasculitis
- Peripheral neuropathy (increased risk in alcoholics, diabetics)
- Blood dyscrasias
- Nausea, vomiting

SPECIAL NURSING CONSIDERATIONS:

- Monitor CBC, liver function tests baseline and at least monthly during therapy
- Stop all drugs if liver function abnormalities occur, then add back one at a time to identify offending agent
- Discontinue drug immediately if signs/symptoms of hepatitis occur
- Discontinue drug immediately if sensitivity reaction occurs; can restart at lower dose, but discontinue immediately if hypersensitivity recurs
- Administer pyridoxine hydrochloride concomitantly in alcoholic and diabetic patients to decrease risk of neuropathy
- Baseline ophthalmologic exam; referral and periodic exams if visual changes occur
- ATS/CDC 6-month therapy regime:
  —INH 5 mg/kg (up to 300 mg)
  —Rifampin 10 mg/kg (up to 600 mg)
  —Pyrazinamide 15–30 mg/kg (up to 2 gm) q day X 2 months, then
  —INH, rifampin q d or 2 X/week X 4 months
- ATS/CDC 9-month regime:
  —INH 5 mg/kg (up to 300 mg)
  —Rifampin 10 mg/kg (up to 600 mg) q day X 1–2 months until sputum cultures negative, then
  —INH 15 mg/kg (max 900 mg)
  —Rifampin 10 mg/kg (max 600 mg) q day or 2 X/week X 7–8 months
- Ethambutol added if resistance to INH suspected

PATIENT EDUCATION:
- Report immediately signs/symptoms of hepatitis (headache, weakness, malaise, anorexia, nausea, vomiting)
- Report any visual changes immediately
- Need for long-term therapy

Itraconazole

BRAND NAME:
- Sporanox

ACTION:
- Antifungal

INDICATIONS:
- Oral treatment of histoplasmosis and blastomycosis Investigational: invasive aspergillosis, coccidioidomycosis, sporotrichosis, cryptococcosis, candidiasis

CONTRAINDICATIONS:
- Known hypersensitivity to the drug;
- Breast-feeding mothers; use with caution when benefit outweighs risk in pregnant women, and in children

DOSAGE:
- 200 mg q d in patients with normal immune responsiveness
- 200 mg bid in patients with AIDS, other immu- nosuppressive states

ADMINISTRATION:
• Oral, with food

DRUG INTERACTIONS:
• Isoniazid, rifampin, phenobarbitol, carbamazepine, phenytoin: increases itraconazole metabolism and decreases drug effects; may need to increase dose of itraconazole
• Phenytoin, cyclosporine, oral hypoglycemics, warfarin, digoxin, terfenadine, astemizole: itraconazole may slow drug metabolism and increase toxicity of these agents
• Terfenadine, possibly astemizole: possible LIFE-THREATENING ventricular tachycardia. AVOID CONCURRENT USE.

ADVERSE EFFECTS:
• At doses of 400 mg/day, occurring in 5–10% of patients
  —Nausea and vomiting Hypokalemia
  —increased LFTs (aminotransferase)
• At doses of 600 mg/day
  —Hypertension, severe hypokalemia
  —Adrenal insufficiency, rhabdomyolysis
  —Rarely, hepatitis, toxic epidermal necrolysis

SPECIAL NURSING CONSIDERATIONS:
• Monitor serum potassium periodically during treatment

- Monitor drug levels in patients with severe hepatic insufficiency
- Usual treatment course for disseminated or chronic pulmonary histoplasmosis is at least 12 months. but may be life-time in patients with AIDS
- Usual treatment for blastomycosis is 6–12 months, but may be lifetime in patients with AIDS

PATIENT EDUCATION:
- Take drug with food
- Need for prolonged treatment
- Report nausea/vomiting

Kaolin-Pectin

BRAND NAMES:
- Kaodene, Kaopectate

ACTION:
- Antidiarrheal agent; absorbs and protects mucosa, thus decreasing fluidity of stool

INDICATIONS:
- Temporary relief of diarrhea

CONTRAINDICATIONS:
- Known hypersensitivity

DOSAGE:
- *Adult:* 60–120 mL (regular) or 45–90 mL concentrated suspension after each loose stool X 48 hours

ADMINISTRATION:
- Oral
- Shake well prior to administration

DRUG INTERACTIONS:
- Oral lincomycin: decreases lincomycin absorption; administer kaolin-pectin 2 hours before or 3–4 hours after antibiotic
- Oral digoxin: decreases digoxin absorption: give kaolin-pectin 2 hours after digoxin

ADVERSE EFFECTS:
- Transient constipation

SPECIAL NURSING CONSIDERATIONS:
- Drug is not absorbed from gastrointestinal tract
- Well tolerated

PATIENT EDUCATION:
- Serf-administration
- Notify physician/nurse if diarrhea persists > 48 hours or if fever develops
- Increase oral fluids to 3 L/day

Ketoconazole

BRAND NAME:
- Nizoril

ACTION:
- Antifungal

INDICATIONS:
- Candidiasis (chronic or systemic mucocutaneous), chromomycosis, coccidioidomycosis, histoplasmosis, paracoccidioidomycosis, dermatophyte (severe, cutaneous infections)

CONTRAINDICATIONS:
- Known hypersensitivity, breast-feeding mothers;
- Use with caution when benefit outweighs risk in children or pregnant women

DOSAGE:
- *Adult:* 200 mg q d
- *Children:* 3.3–6.6 mg/kg q d

ADMINISTRATION:
- Oral, take with meals if needed to decrease nausea

DRUG INTERACTIONS:
- Antacids, anticholinergics, cimetidine, ranitidine, other H_2 antagonists, didanosine: decreases

ketoconazole absorption. GIVE THESE DRUGS
2 HOURS AFTER KETOCONAZOLE DOSE
- Isoniazid, rifampin: increases ketoconazole
metabolism: may need to increase
ketoconazole dose

ADVERSE EFFECTS:
- Nausea and vomiting (3–10% of patients)
- *Less common:*
  —Headache, nervousness, dizziness, pruritis
  —Abdominal pain, diarrhea, constipation
  —Increased LFTs, gynecomastia, breast
  tenderness

SPECIAL NURSING CONSIDERATIONS:
- Monitor liver function tests in patients with
hepatic dysfunction or taking other hepatotoxic
drugs
- Drug requires an acid environment to be
absorbed. Approximately 25% of patients with
AIDS may be achlorhydric and require change
to fluconazole or another antifungal azole that
does not require the same gastric acidity.
Alternatively, may dissolve ketoconazole tablet
in 4 mL aqueous solution of 0.2 N hydrochloric
acid; then drug is sipped through a straw to
prevent staining of teeth; swallow with 8 oz.
water.

PATIENT EDUCATION:
- Teach patient to take drug with food to reduce
nausea/vomiting if this occurs

Lamivudine (3TC)

BRAND NAME:
- Investigational agent

ACTION:
- Antiretroviral agent, inhibits the enzyme reverse transcriptase, thus preventing HIV replication

INDICATIONS:
- *Adult:* phase II–III clinical trials in HIV disease (in progress)
- *Children:* phase I–II (in progress)

CONTRAINDICATIONS:
- Unknown

DOSAGE:
- *Adult:* 150–300 mg PO bid
- Per protocol

ADMINISTRATION:
- Oral

DRUG INTERACTIONS:
- Unknown

ADVERSE EFFECTS:
- Neutropenia, macrocytosis without anemia
- Increased serum amylase
- Peripheral neuropathy

SPECIAL NURSING CONSIDERATIONS:
- Toxicity profile milder than for zidovudine
- Drug is well tolerated in asymptomatic patients as well as those with CD^4 counts < 200/mm³
- NIH study investigating efficacy in HIV-infected children who have previously received little or no prior antiretroviral therapy. For further information, call (301) 402-1387
- Manufacturer: Glaxo Pharmaceuticals (1-800-334-0089)

PATIENT EDUCATION:
- Drug self-administration per protocol

Leucovorin
Calcium Citrovorum Factor
(Folinic Acid)

BRAND NAME:
- Wellcovorin

ACTION:
- Antidote for methotrexate and other folic acid antagonists; circumvents biochemical enzyme blockade, permitting RNA and DNA synthesis

INDICATIONS:
- In conjunction with high- and medium-dose methotrexate to decrease hematologic toxicity

CONTRAINDICATIONS:
- Known hypersensitivity
- Undiagnosed anemia

DOSAGE:
- As rescue for methotrexate: 10 mg/m^2 IV/PO q 6 hours X 6–8 doses, beginning 24 hours after methotrexate

ADMINISTRATION:
- Oral: tablet, oral solution or parenteral form can be given orally
- IM/IV: following methotrexate drug MUST BE GIVEN EXACTLY ON TIME. Drug must be on hand before methotrexate given

DRUG INTERACTIONS:
- Phenobarbital, phenytoin, pyrimidone: large doses of leucovorin may counteract anti-eleptic effects; monitor serum drug levels and increase dose of anticonvulsant

ADVERSE EFFECTS:
- *Uncommon:*
  —Allergy (facial flushing, itching)
- *Rare:*
  —Nausea

SPECIAL NURSING CONSIDERATIONS:
- Leucovorin calcium powder for oral solution is reconstituted with 21–23% alcohol aromatic

elixir; monitor closely or use alternative form in substance abusers or if alcohol should be avoided

PATIENT EDUCATION:
- Administer dose exactly on time as prescribed
- Notify physician/nurse if unable to take drug

Loperamide

BRAND NAME:
- Imodium

ACTION:
- Antidiarrheal agent; inhibits peristalsis, slowing intestinal motility, increasing stool bulk and viscosity

INDICATIONS:
- Temporary relief of diarrhea

CONTRAINDICATIONS:
- Acute diarrhea caused by mucosal-penetrating organisms *(Shigella, E. coli)*
- Diarrhea due to pseudomembranous colitis
- Known hypersensitivity
- Use cautiously in patients with acute ulcerative colitis, pregnancy, or in nursing mothers

DOSAGE:
* *Adult:* 4 mg PO, followed by 2 mg PO after each unformed stool (max 16 mg if under direction of physician, 8 mg if self-medicating/24 hours)

ADMINISTRATION:
* Oral

DRUG INTERACTIONS:
* None

ADVERSE EFFECTS:
* Nausea, vomiting, diarrhea, abdominal pain and distention
* Drowsiness, fatigue, dizziness
* Rarely, rash

SPECIAL NURSING CONSIDERATIONS:
* 2–3 X more potent than diphenoxylate (Lomotil), with fewer adverse reactions
* Risk of development of megacolon when used in patients with ulcerative colitis; discontinue drug if abdominal distention occurs
* Reduces electrolyte and fluid loss
* Assess history of ulcerative colitis

PATIENT EDUCATION:
* Notify physician/nurse:
  —If diarrhea doesn't resolve in 48 hours or if fever, abdominal pain occur
  —Report rash, abdominal distention immediately
  —Increase PO fluids to 3 L/day

Lorazepam

BRAND NAME:
- Ativan

ACTION:
- Anxiolytic (benzodiazepine) agent; causes anxiety reduction, muscle relaxation, and some anticonvulsant effect

INDICATIONS:
- Anxiety
- Preoperative sedation
- Used in combination as an antiemetic agent for cancer chemotherapy

CONTRAINDICATIONS:
- Known hypersensitivity
- Acute narrow angle glaucoma
- Pregnancy and nursing mothers
- Depressive neuroses, psychotic reaction
- Use cautiously if liver or renal impairment,pulmonary disease

DOSAGE:
- *Adults:*
  —Oral: 1–6 mg/day in divided doses (max 10 mg/day)
  —IM: 0.044 mg/kg (up to 2 mg) as initial dose

—IV: 0.044 mg/kg (upto 2 mg) given 15–20 minutes prior to surgery; up to 1.4 mg/m^2 given 30 minutes prior to chemotherapy

ADMINISTRATION:
- Oral dose may be given with food to decrease stomach distress
- IM: administer deep IM into large muscle mass
- IV: IV push or IV bolus over 15 minutes
- NEVER GIVE DRUG INTRA-ARTERIALLY

DRUG INTERACTIONS:
- Alcohol, CNS depressants: increases CNS depression; avoid or monitor closely
- Oral contraceptives, isoniazid, ketoconazole: increase lorazepam serum levels; monitor for sedation
- Digoxin: decrease digoxin excretion; monitor digoxin level and adjust dose

ADVERSE EFFECTS:
- Drowsiness, fatigue, lethargy, headache, vivid dreams
- Nausea, vomiting, weight gain. increased liver function tests
- Amnesia, sedation lasting ≥ 8 hours
- Bradycardia, hypotension
  Rash, pruritis

SPECIAL NURSING CONSIDERATIONS:
- Has amnesic effect so useful as antiemetic agent for cancer chemotherapy

- May cause psychologic dependence (addiction) so use cautiously in substance abuse patients

PATIENT EDUCATION
- Risk of psychological dependence
- Use only for reason prescribed
- Avoid activities requiring mental alertness (driving car, operating heavy machinery)
- Change position slowly while taking the drug
- Report rash

Megestrol Acetate

BRAND NAME:
- Megace

ACTION:
- Synthetic progestin; alters malignant cell environment removing stimulus to proliferate; antagonizes cachexin directly or indirectly and appears to stimulate appetite and weight gain

INDICATIONS:
- Palliative treatment of breast and endometrial cancers
- AIDS-related anorexia, cachexia, weight loss > 10% of baseline

CONTRAINDICATIONS:
- Known hypersensitivity
- Pregnancy

DOSAGE:
- *Adult:*
  - —40 mg PO qid to 800 mg/day in divided doses
  - —Optimal dosing for cachexia may be 800 mg/day (Loprinzi, Jensen, Burnham et al, 1992)

ADMINISTRATION:
- Oral, tablets or liquid

DRUG INTERACTIONS:
- None

ADVERSE EFFECTS:
- Deep vein thrombosis (6% of patients)
- Nausea, vomiting
- Break through vaginal bleeding
- Decreased libido and sexual dysfunction in males

SPECIAL NURSING CONSIDERATIONS:
- Weight appears to be due to increased fat stores not water gain
- May take 1–2 months
- Associated with improvement in mood

PATIENT EDUCATION:
- Report pain in calf, erythema. shortness of breath, chest pain immediately
- Breakthrough vaginal bleeding may occur

Meperidine Hydrochloride

BRAND NAME:
- Demerol

ACTION:
- Synthetic narcotic analgesic

INDICATIONS:
- Moderate to severe acute pain
- Preoperative sedation
- Used to stop/prevent rigors associated with fever due to amphotericin B or blood transfusion sensitization

CONTRAINDICATIONS:
- Known hypersensitivity
- Sulfite hypersensitivity
- Use with caution in atrial flutter, other supraventricular tachycardias, hepatic or renal dysfunction, severe CNS depression, head Injury

DOSAGE:
- Oral; 50–150 mg q 3–4 hours
- IM: 50–150 mg q 3–4 hours
- IV: 50–100 mg IVP
- SC: 50–150 mg q 3–4 hours
- Dose reduce if renal or hepatic dysfunction exists

Memory Bank for HIV Medications

ADMINISTRATION:
- Oral, IM, IV, or SC
- Drug should be administered with caution ifused long-term

DRUG INTERACTIONS:
- Isoniazid (NIH): increase INH toxicity; monitor patient closely
- Alcohol, CNS depressants: increase CNS depression; monitor closely
- Aspirin, acetaminophen: increase analgesia; use to advantage
- Hydrozyzine: increase analgesic effect; use to advantage
- Injection incompatible with solutions containing aminophylline, barbiturates, ephedrine sulfate, heparin sodium, hydrocortisone sodium succinate, methicillin sodium, methylprednisolone sodium succinate, morphine sulfate, tetracycline
- Naloxone: antagonist; use to reverse overdose or respiratory depression

ADVERSE EFFECTS:
- Normeperidine toxicity: CNS stimulation; monitor patient receiving frequent or high doses closely
- Drowsiness, sedation, mood changes, miosis
- Constipation, ileus
- Nausea, vomiting, dry mouth

- Orthostatic hypotension
- Urinary retention, spasm, urgency
- Rarely, respiratory depression

SPECIAL NURSING CONSIDERATIONS:
- Active metabolite normeperidine can accumulate with chronic use; it is a potent CNS stimulant causing seizures, agitation, irritability, nervousness, myoclonus
- Oral meperidine (50 mg) is equivelant to acetaminophen 650 mg or aspirin 650 mg in terms of analgesic effect
- Sedative and euphoric effects greater than morphine
- Not used for long-term management of chronic pain because of short duration of action, severe risk of neurotoxicity, and decreased bioavailability
- Give smallest effective dose to prevent development of tolerance, physical dependency

PATIENT EDUCATION:
- Avoid driving car, operating machinery while taking drug
- Avoid concurrent alcohol
- Report rash, nausea, vomiting
- Report if no bowel movement in 2 days
- Change position slowly

Methadone Hydrochloride

BRAND NAME:
- Dolophine

ACTION:
- Narcotic analgesic

INDICATIONS:
- Moderate to severe pain
- Prevention of abstinence syndrome in heroin detoxification and maintenance programs

CONTRAINDICATIONS:
- Known hypersensitivity
- Nursing mothers
- Use with caution in pregnancy, patients with hepatic or renal dysfunction, CNS depression, respiratory depression, head injury

DOSAGE:
- Oral:
  —5–20 mg q 6–8 hours, or more for severe cancer pain
  —Maintenance dose adjusted to prevent abstinence syndrome
- SC, IM: 2.5–10 mg q 3–4 hours

ADMINISTRATION:
- Oral tablet, oral liquid given in juice for patients receiving detoxification or maintenance therapy
- Round-the-clock dosing, not prn, necessary to control/prevent chronic cancer pain

DRUG INTERACTIONS:
- Isoniazid (NIH): increase INH toxicity; monitor patient closely
- Alcohol, CNS depressants: increase CNS depression; monitor closely
- Aspirin, acetaminophen: increase analgesia; use to advantage
- Hydrozyzine: increase analgesic effect; use to advantage
- Desipramine: may increase serum desipramine level; assess closely for toxicity
- Rifampin, rifabutin: increase metabolism of methadone causing possible drug withdrawal symptoms; use together cautiously and increase methadone dose as needed
- Injection incompatible with solutions containing aminophylline, barbiturates, ephedrine sulfate, heparin sodium, hydrocortisone sodium succinate, methicillin sodium, methylprednisolone sodium succinate, morphine sulfate, tetracycline
- Naloxone: antagonist; use to reverse overdose or respiratory depression

ADVERSE EFFECTS:
- Drowsiness, sedation, mood changes, miosis
- Constipation, ileus
- Nausea, vomiting, dry mouth
- Orthostatic hypotension
- Urinary retention, spasm, urgency
- Rarely, respiratory depression

SPECIAL NURSING CONSIDERATIONS:
- Equianalgesic oral dose is 2 X parenteral dose
- Additive effect when combined with acetaminophen or aspirin
- May produce similar or slightly greater respiratory depression than equivalent doses of morphine
- Give smallest effective dose to prevent development of tolerance, physical dependency

PATIENT EDUCATION:
- Avoid driving car, operating machinery while taking drug
- Avoid concurrent alcohol
- Report rash, nausea, vomiting
- Report if no bowel movement in 2 days
- Change position slowly

Methotrexate Sodium

BRAND NAMES:
- Amethopterin, Folex, Mexate

ACTION:
- Antimetabolite antineoplastic agent; inhibits folic acid synthesis, preventing RNA and DNA synthesis in rapidly proliferating cells

INDICATIONS:
- Lymphoma

CONTRAINDICATIONS:
- Known hypersensitivity
- Nursing mothers
- Renal failure
- Pregnancy

DOSAGE:
- IV:
  —Low: 10–50 mg/m^2
  —Medium: 100–500 mg/m^2 with leukovorin rescue
  —High: > 500 mg/m^2 with leukovorin rescue 24 hours after drug administration
- IT: 10–15 mg/m^2
- IM: 25 mg/m^2

ADMINISTRATION:

- IV low: IVP
- IV medium: in 100–250 mL IV solution administered over 20 minutes–1 hour
- IT: drug must be reconstituted aseptically with
  preservative-free diluent
- IV: High doses must be mixed with preservative-free diluent; infuse over 3 or more hours;
  urine must be alkalinized, and hydration given
  to ensure urinary output of at least 100 mL/hour
- USE SAFE CHEMOTHERAPY HANDLING
  PRECAUTIONS (see Appendix I)

DRUG INTERACTIONS:

- Protein-bound drugs (aspirin, sulfonamides,
  sulfonylureas, phenytoin, tetracycline,
  chloramphenicol); increased toxicity; give
  together cautiously and monitor patient closely
- NSAIDs (nonsteroidal anti-inflammatory drugs
  (e.g., indomethacin, ketoprofen): increased and
  prolonged methotrexate (MTX)levels; DO NOT
  administer concurrently with high doses of MTX:
  monitor patients closely who are receiving
  moderate or low dose MTX
- Co-trimoxazole: increased MTX serum level; do
  not use concurrently
- Pyrimethamine: increased MTX serum level; do
  not use concurrently

ADVERSE EFFECTS:

- Nausea, vomiting (rare with low, mild with
  medium dose)

- Stomatitis, diarrhea
- Photosensitivity
- Renal failure
- Bone marrow suppression, nadir 7–9 days after drug administration
- Dizziness, blurred vision, malaise when given ITor after cranial radiation

SPECIAL NURSING CONSIDERATIONS:
- Calcium leukovorin "rescues" normal cells, preventing bone marrow toxicity, mucositis
- Monitor baseline and prechemo BUN, serum creatinine, CBC prior to drug administration
- Hold treatment if stomatitis or diarrhea occur
- Monitor liver function tests baseline and periodically during treatment
- Administer antiemetics at least prior to initial dose
- Given in combination with other agents (e.g., M-BACOD)
- USE SAFE CHEMOTHERAPY HANDLING PRECAUTIONS

PATIENT EDUCATION:
- Report mouth sores or diarrhea immediately
- Need for frequent blood tests
- Oral hygiene regimen PC and HS
- Avoid strong sunlight; use sun protection factor (SPF) 15
- Report blurred vision, dizziness if receiving drug IT

Methylphenidate Hydrochloride

BRAND NAMES:
- Ritalin, Ritalin SR

ACTION:
- Mild central nervous system (CNS) stimulant; probably activates brain stem arousal system and cortex

INDICATIONS:
- Attention deficit disorders, narcolepsy
- May be used to increase energy in patients with advanced HIV disease

CONTRAINDICATIONS:
- Patients with marked anxiety, tension, agitation,glaucoma, Tourette's syndrome
- Known hypersensitivity

DOSAGE:
- 5–10 mg PO tid

ADMINISTRATION:
- Available in 5, 10, 20 mg tablets and in 20 mg sustained-release tablets (Ritalin-SR)
- Give 30 minutes before meals

DRUG INTERACTIONS:
- Guanethidine: decreases hypotensive effect
- Coumarin anticoagulants, anticonvulsants, tricyclic antidepressants: methyl phenidate decreases drug metabolism; decrease drug dose as needed

ADVERSE EFFECTS:
- Nervousness, insomnia
- Hypersensitivity (rash, urticaria, arthralgia, fever; rarely, thrombocytopenia purpura, exfoliative dermatitis)
- Anorexia
- Headache, dizziness

SPECIAL NURSING CONSIDERATIONS:
- Often reverses apathy
- Not effective in severe dementia
- Assess for increased CNS stimulation and seizure potential (hyperreflexia, muscle twitching, euphoria, confusion)
- Hallucinations, hypertension, mydriasis
- Discontinue drug if trial is ineffective

PATIENT EDUCATION:
- Take drug in the morning to decrease insomnia
- Report agitation, tremors, or change in condition

Metronidazole Hydrochloride

BRAND NAME:
- Flagyl

ACTION:
- Antibiotic with action against bacteria and protozoa; disrupts DNA, causing cell death

INDICATIONS:
- Gram-positive (e.g., *Clostridium),* gram-negative (e.g., *Bacteroides),* and protozoa (e.g., *Trichomonas, Giardia)*

CONTRAINDICACTIONS:
- Known hypersensitivity
- Nursing mothers
- Pregnancy
- Use with caution if blood dyscrasia, CNS disorders/dysfunction, hepatic dysfunction, alcoholism

DOSAGE:
- *Adult:*
  —Oral: 250–750 mg PO tid X 7–10 days or single dose of 2 gm PO (trichomoniasis)
  —IV: loading dose of 15 mg/kg IV, then maintenance dose of 7.5 mg/kg IV q 6 hours (max 4 gm/day)

ADMINISTRATION:
- IV dose: administer diluted drug over 30–60 minutes
- DO NOT USE ALUMINUM NEEDLES

DRUG INTERACTIONS:
- Coumarin anticoagulants: increases anticoagulant effect. Avoid concurrent use if possible; otherwise, monitor prothrombin time closely and decrease anticoagulant drug dose needed
- Alcohol: inhibits alcohol metabolism, causing a disulfiram-like reaction (flushing, headache, nausea, vomiting, abdominal cramps, diaphoresis). Avoid alcohol, alcohol-containing medications for > 48 hours after last metronidazole dose
- Disulfiram: causes acute psychoses and confusion. Avoid concurrent use and separate use by 2 weeks
- Phenobarbital, phenytoin: decrease metronidazole activity. Monitor effectiveness and increase metronidazole dose as needed
- Cimetidine: increases metronidazole levels with potential for increased toxicity. Avoid concurrent administration

ADVERSE EFFECTS:
- Nausea, anorexia, dry mouth, metallic taste
- Vomiting, diarrhea
- Peripheral neuropathy

- Rash, urticaria, pruritis
- Dysuria, dark or reddish-brown urine color
- Phlebitis at IV site

SPECIAL NURSING CONSIDERATIONS:
- Fungal superinfection may occur on mucous membranes (oral thrush, vaginal candidiasis)

PATIENT EDUCATION:
- Avoid alcohol
- Stop drug and report numbness, stingling of hands, feet
- Report rash, itching
- Drug may cause urine to be temporarily darkened in color
- Increase oral fluids to 2–3 L/day
- Report candidal infections of mucous membranes

Miconazole

BRAND NAME:
- Monistat IV

ACTION:
- Antifungal agent; destroys fungal cell membrane, killing organism

INDICATIONS:
- Severe fungal infections (e.g., coccidioidomycosis, candidiasis; cryptococcosis)

CONTRAINDICATIONS:
- Known hypersensitivity

DOSAGE:
- *Adult:*
  —IV: coccidioidomycosis: 1.8–3.6 gm/day X 320+ weeks; cryptococcosis: 1.2–2.4 gm/day X 3–12+ weeks; candidiasis: 600 mg–1.8 gm/day X 1–20+ weeks
  —IT: refer to protocol, usually 20 mg q 1–2 days, or q 3–7 days if given by lumbar puncture
  —Intravesicai: 200 mg in dilute solution 2—4 X per day or by continual bladder irrigation •
  Children (1–12 years):
  —Total daily doses 20–40 mg/kg (dose max is 15 mg/kg)

ADMINISTRATION:
- IV: dilute 200 mg of drug in at least 200 mL of IV solution, and infuse over 2 hours
- CARDLOPULMONARY ARREST AND/OR ANAPHYLAXIS HAS OCCURRED WHEN INFUSED TOO RAPIDLY

DRUG INTERACTIONS:
- Coumarin anticoagulants: increased prothrombin time. Monitor patient closely and decrease anticoagulant dose accordingly
- Norfloxacin: may increase antifungal action
- Oral sulfonylureas: increased hypoglycemia effect. Monitor blood glucose and decrease dose of oral sulfonylurea
- Rifampin or rifampin plus isoniazid: decreased miconazole' levels, especially if isoniazid taken as well. Increase miconazole dose
- Phenytoin: may have altered serum levels of phenytoin or miconazole. Monitor serum levels of each and adjust dosages accordingly
- Cyclosporine: increased cyclosporine serum level. Monitor serum level and decrease cyclosporine dose accordingly

ADVERSE EFFECTS:
- Allergic reaction, including anaphylaxis with tachycardia, arrhythmias
- Phlebitis, pruritis, rash
- Nausea, vomiting, diarrhea, anorexia
- Headache, blurred vision, dizziness, increased libido

SPECIAL NURSING CONSIDERATIONS:
- Drug is suspended in castor oil base, which stimulates allergic response. First dose should be administered in a hospital setting with resuscitation equipment readily available

Drug Profiles

- Monitor hemoglobin/hematocrit, serum electro-lytes, and lipids, as changes may occur during treatment

PATIENT EDUCATION:
- Report immediately: nausea, generalized itching, crampy abdominal pain, chest tightness, anxiety, agitation, sense of impending doom, wheeze, dizziness

Morphine Sulfate

BRAND NAMES:
- Astramorph, Duramorph, MS Contin, MSIR, Oramorph, Roxanol

ACTION:
- Synthetic narcotic analgesic

INDICATIONS:
- Moderate to severe acute pain
- Preoperative sedation

CONTRAINDICATIONS:
- Known hypersensitivity
- Sulfite hypersensitivity
- Use with caution in patients with hepatic or renal dysfunction, severe CNS depression, head injury, respiratory depression, hypothyroidism

DOSAGE:
- Oral:
  10–60 mg PO q 3–4 hours titrated to pain
  10–240 mg sustained release q 8–12 hours,
  titrated to pain
- Rectal: 10–60 mg q 4 hours
- SC, IM: 4–15 mg q 3–4 hours
- IV: 1–100 mg/hour or higher as needed to
  relieve severe pain
- Intrathecal (IT): 1/10 epidural dose
- Epidural: 5 mg q 24 hours

ADMINISTRATION:
- Oral, rectal, SC, IM, IV, IT, epidural
- Preservative-free preparations must be used for
  IT or epidural routes
- Round-the-clock dosing, not prn, necessary to
  control/prevent chronic cancer pain

DRUG INTERACTIONS:
- Isoniazid (INH): increase INH toxicity; monitor
  patient closely
- Alcohol, CNS depressants: increase CNS
  depression; monitor closely
- Aspirin, acetaminophen: increase analgesia;
  use to advantage
- Hydroxyzine: increase analgesic effect; use to
  advantage

- Injection incompatible with solutions containing aminophylline, barbiturates, ephedrine sulfate, heparin sodium, hydrocortisone sodium succinate, methicillin sodium, methylpredniso-lone sodium succinate, morphine sulfate, tetracycline
- Naloxone: antagonist; use to reverse overdose or respiratory depression

ADVERSE EFFECTS:
- Constipation
- Drowsiness, sedation, mood changes
- Hypotension, brachycardia
- Respiratory depression
- Urinary spasm, retention
- Tolerance and dependency

SPECIAL NURSING CONSIDERATIONS:
- Begin morphine therapy using immediate release oral preparations and increase dose to control pain; once optimal dose identified, convert to sustained-release formulation by dividing 24-hour total morphine dose by 2, giving 2 (q 12 hour) doses
- Oral to parenteral dose is 3–6 to 1 (equianalgesic dose)
- Tolerance to respiratory depressive effects occurs with continued drug use
- Highly concentrated formulation available for use in continuous infusion ambulatory pumps

- Give smallest effective dose to relieve pain to prevent development of tolerance and physical dependency
- Constipation must be prevented by regular bowel regime (stool softener, hydration, fiber, cathartic as needed)
- Withdrawal symptoms may occur if round-the clock dosing is interrupted (restlessness, lacrimation, rhinorrhea)

PATIENT EDUCATION:
- Avoid driving car, operating machinery while taking drug
- Avoid concurrent alcohol
- Report rash, nausea, vomiting
- Report if no bowel movement in 2 days
- Change position slowly
- Follow bowel regime

Mupirocin 2%

BRAND NAME:
- Bactroban

ACTION:
- Antibiotic

INDICATIONS:
- Skin infections:
  —Impetigo *(Staphylococcus aureus,* folliculitis, group B-hemolytic *Streptococcus)*
  —Furuculosis
- Nasal infection with *S. aureus,* including methicillin-resistant *S. aureus*

CONTRAINDICATIONS:
- Patients with burns
- Hypersensitivity
- Use in pregnancy only when benefit > risk
- Use in breast-feeding mothers
- Use with caution in patients with renal dysfunction

DOSAGE:
- Small amount applied to affected area tid, may cover with sterile gauze

ADMINISTRATION:
- If no improvement within 3–5 days, reevaluate
- Impetigo: 1–2 week treatment

DRUG INTERACTIONS:
- None known

ADVERSE EFFECTS:
- *Rare:*
  —Burning, stinging, pain pruritis, erythema, rash, dry skin, increased exudate
  —May develop overgrowth of nonsusceptible micro-organism, e.g., fungi

SPECIAL NURSING CONSIDERATIONS:
- Prolonged or repeated application to damaged skin (burns) can lead to absorption of toxic amounts

PATIENT EDUCATION:
- Do not apply to eye
- Self-application technique

Naproxen

BRAND NAMES:
- Naprosyn, Anaprox

ACTION:
- Nonsteroidal anti-inflammatory agent; has antiinflammatory, analgesic, and antipyretic actions, probably through prostaglandin inhibition

INDICATIONS:
- Mild to moderate pain
- Osteoarthritis
- Has been used to reduce/prevent fever

CONTRAINDICATIONS:
- Known hypersensitivity to naproxen
- Sensitivity to aspirin or other nonsteroidal antiinflammatory drugs
- Pregnancy, or in nursing mothers only when benefit outweighs risk

- Asthma with nasal polyps
- Use with caution, if at all, in history of pepticulcer disease

DOSAGE:
- *Adult:* initial dose of 500 mg PO, then 250 mg q 6–8 hours prn, or 250–375 mg tid
- Max dose total 1.25 gm

ADMINISTRATION:
- Available in 250, 375 and 500 mg tablets and oral suspension 125 mg/5 mL
- Administer drug with meals, milk, or aluminumor magnesium-containing antacids

DRUG INTERACTIONS:
- Methotrexate: increases methotrexate serum levels; avoid concurrent use
- Probenecid: increases naproxen serum level; monitor for toxicity and decrease dose
- Salicylates: increases bleeding; do not use concurrently
- Warfarin: increases bleeding risk; use together with caution if at all

ADVERSE EFFECTS:
- Renal dysfunction
- Constipation, heartburn, abdominal pain, nausea

- Elevated liver function tests
- Reactivate latent peptic ulcer, or may cause peptic ulcers in patients without a history of ulcers
- Rash, pruritis
- Headache, drowsiness. dizziness, tinnitus
- Rarely, visual disturbances
- Prolonged bleeding time

SPECIAL NURSING CONSIDERATIONS:
- Monitor renal, liver function studies baseline and periodically in patients receiving drug long-term
- Refer for ophthalmologic exam if patient develops visual disturbances
- Maximum therapeutic effect may take 2–4 weeks
- Naproxen (Naprosyn) 250 mg equivalent to naproxen sodium (Anaprox) 275 mg, 500 mg equivalent to naproxen sodium 550 mg; do not take both drugs at same time

PATIENT EDUCATION:
- Report coughing up blood, black stools, dizziness immediately
- Report any visual disturbances immediately

Norfloxacin

BRAND NAME:
- Noroxin

ACTION:
- Broad-spectrum quinolone antibiotic agent; prevents bacterial DNA synthesis. Active against most gram-negative and some gram-positive organisms

INDICATIONS:
- Urinary tract infections (UTI)
- Uncomplicated urethral and cervical gonorrhea
- Has been used to treat gastroenteritis caused by suscepffible organisms *(Shigella)*

CONTRAINDICATIONS:
- Known hypersensitivity to drug
- Known hypersensitivity to other quinolone antibiotics
- Pregnancy, nursing mothers
- Children
- Use with caution in seizure and CNS disorders

DOSAGE:
- UTI: 400 mg bid X 7–10 days (uncomplicated and X 10–21 days (complicated)
- Gonorrhea: single 800 mg oral dose
- Max dose 800 mg/day
- Modify dose in renal dysfunction

ADMINISTRATION:
- Oral; give with full glass of water 1 hour before or 2 hours after food

DRUG INTERACTIONS:
- Aluminum- or magnesium-containing antacids: decrease norfloxacin absorption; avoid concurrent use or administer 2 hours apart
- Antifungal drugs (e.g., amphotericin, ketoconazole): may be synergistic
- Warfarin: may increase prothrombin time (PT); monitor PT closely and reduce coumadin dose
- Nitrofurantoin: antagonism; do not use together
- Theophylline: increase theophylline level; monitor serum drug level and reduce dose

ADVERSE EFFECTS:
- *Uncommon:*
    - —Crystalluria: increases BUN, serum creatinine
    - —Nausea, vomiting, diarrhea, abdominal pain
    - —Headache, dizziness, lightheadedness
    - —Eosinophilia, rash, pruritis; rare anaphylaxis
    - —Arthralgia, myalgia

SPECIAL NURSING CONSIDERATIONS:
- As effective as co-trimoxazole in treating UTIs but with fewer side effects
- Causes arthropathy in immature animals, so drug should not be used in children

PATIENT EDUCATiON:
- Take tablet with full glass of water, 1 hour before or 2 hours after food
- Change position slowly
- If dizziness occurs, do not drive a vehicle or operate machinery
- Avoid excessive sunlight exposure, caffeine intake
- Stop drug and notify physician if rash develops

Nortriptyline

BRAND NAMES:
- Aventyl, Pamelor

ACTION:
- Tricyclic antidepressant

INDICATIONS:
- Relief of depression

CONTRAINDICATIONS:
- Known hypersensitivity
- Seizure disorder
- Benign prostate hypertrophy
- Immediately following acute myocardial infarction

- Within 2 weeks of, or concurrently with, a monoamine oxidase (MAO) inhibitor drug
- Use cautiously in patients with urine retention, narrow-angle glaucoma, hyperthyroidism, hepatic dysfunction, suicidal ideation

DOSAGE:
- *Adult*: oral: 75–100 mg q d in divided or single dose at bedtime
- Dose may be increased to maximum 150 mg/day

ADMINISTRATION:
- Administer as single bedtime dose since drug has long half-life, or can give in 3–4 divided doses

DRUG INTERACTIONS:
- Cimetidine: increases nortriptyline levels, increasing toxicity; monitor patient closely for toxicity
- Barbiturates: may decrease nortriptyline levels; monitor for response and increase dose as needed
- CNS depressants (alcohol, sedatives, hypnotics): increase CNS depression; use together cautiously
- Coumadin: increases prothrombin time; monitor patient closely, decrease coumadin dose as needed

- Monoamine oxidase (MAO) inhibitors: hyperpyretic crisis, convulsions, death; avoid concurrent, and separate use by 2 weeks
- Quinidine: increases nortriptyline levels; monitor for toxicity
- Sympathomimetic drugs (epinephrine, amphetamines): increases hypertension; AVOID concurrent use

ADVERSE EFFECTS:
- Drowsiness, weakness, lethargy, fatigue
- Dry mouth, anorexia, nausea/vomiting
- Elevated liver function tests (uncommon)
- Rash, urticaria, photosensitivity

SPECIAL NURSING CONSIDERATIONS:
- Antidepressant effect may take 2 weeks or longer
- Adjuvant analgesic useful in cancer and other types of pain; improves sleep as well
- When discontinued, drug should be withdrawn gradually. Abrupt withdrawal may result in anxiety, malaise, dizziness, nausea/vomiting
- Some preparations contain soduim bisulfite which can cause hypersensitivity reactions. Check drug ingredients and assess patient allergy
- Monitor baseline and periodic liver function tests during therapy

PATIENT EDUCATION:
- Avoid alcohol ingestion, especially if depressed or suicidal
- Take drug as a single dose at bedtime
- Avoid sunlight, or wear sunblock and protective clothes
- Avoid driving a car if drowsy

Nystatin

BRAND NAMES:
- Mycostatin, Nilstat

ACTION:
- Antifungal agent; destroys cell membrane killing yeast and fungi, especially *Candida*

INDICATIONS:
- Candidal infections of mucous membranes

CONTRAINDICATIONS:
- Known hypersensitivity
- Systemic infections

DOSAGE:
- Oral (for treatment of oral or intestinal candidiasis): 500,000–1 million units tid; continue therapy for 48 hours after clinical remission to prevent recurrence
- Powder: topical for candidal rash infections
- Vaginal: 100,000 units as vaginal tablet, inserted into vagina q d or bid X 14 days

ADMINISTRATION:
- Oral suspension:
  —Rinse mouth with oral hygiene solution to clean food debris
  —Hold suspension in mouth and swish for 1–2 minutes, then swallow or spit solution
  —Do not rinse mouth or eat for 15–30 minutes

DRUG INTERACTIONS:
- None (drug not absorbed)

ADVERSE EFFECTS:
- Infrequent
- Nausea, vomiting, diarrhea

SPECIAL NURSING CONSIDERATIONS:
- May be inadequate treatment for many HIV patients, so often ketoconazole or fluconazole is used instead
- Can freeze oral suspension in medicine cups, so easier to administer if patient has stomatitis
- Vaginal suppositories may be sucked, as this increases mucosal contact with drug for oral candidiasis

PATIENT EDUCATION:
- Self-administration

Octreotide Acetate

BRAND NAME:
- Sandostatin

ACTION:
- Analogue of natural hormone somatostatin, and suppresses serotonin and gastroenteropancreatic peptides, gastrin, vasoactive intestinal peptide (VIP), insulin, glucagon, secretin, pancreatic polypeptide, and growth hormone

INDICATIONS:
- Control of symptoms of metastatic carcinoid, and vasoactive intestinal peptide-secreting tumors (watery diarrhea)
- Is used experimentally in management of diarrhea related to cryptosporidium infection

CONTRAINDICATIONS:
- Pregnant or breast-feeding mothers unless benefits outweigh risks

DOSAGE:
- 50 μg SC q 8 hours X 48 hours; if no response, increase stepwise to 500 μg q 8 hours

ADMINISTRATION:
• SC or IV

DRUG INTERACTIONS:
• None known
• Drug may decrease absorption of other oral drugs from GI tract

ADVERSE EFFECTS:
• May enhance formation of gallstones (15–20% of patients)
• *Infrequent:*
  —Constipation, hepatitis, rectal spasm, cholelithiasis
  —Hair loss, pruritis, rash
  —Shortness of breath, congestive heart failure, chest pain
  —Anxiety, depression, forgetfulness

SPECIAL NURSING CONSIDERATIONS:
• In one study, 42% of patients responded with decreased diarrhea

PATIENT EDUCATION:
• Subcutaneous injection technique
• Subcutaneous site rotation
• To report any changes in condition to doctor or nurse

Ofloxacin

BRAND NAME:
• Floxin

ACTION:
• Quinolone broad-spectrum antibiotic;
  bacteriocidal through unclear mechanism

INDICATIONS:
• Infections caused by susceptible organisms of
  the pulmonary system (pneumonia, exacer-
  bated chronic bronchitis), prostate, urinary tract,
  skin; and gonorrhea, *Chlamydia* infections,
  urethritis, cervicitis

CONTRAINDICATIONS:
• Known hypersensitivity to drug or other
  quinolone antibiotics
• Pregnant women
• Nursing mothers
• Children < 18 years old

DOSAGE:
Normal Renal Function:
• UTI, URI
  —200–400 mg q 12 hours X 3–7 days (cystitis)
  to 10 days (lower repiratory tract infections,
  complicated UTI)
• Prostatitis
  —300 mg q 12 hours X 6+ weeks

- Skin and skin structures
  —400 mg q 12 hours X 10 days
- Gonorrhea —400 mg X 1
- Chlamydia, mixed urethral and cervical infection
  —300 mg q 12 hours X 5–7 days
- Decrease dose and/or administration frequency
  if renal insufficiency exists

ADMINISTRATION:
- Oral (IV not commercially available in United
  States)
- Do not administer with food

DRUG INTERACTIONS:
- Antacids, sucralfate, metal cations (e.g., iron,
  zinc), multivitamins containing iron: decrease
  absorption; take 2 hours apart from drug
- Warfarin: increases prothrombin time (PT);
  monitor PT closely and adjust coumadin dose
- Theophylline: increased theophylline level;
  monitor closely and adjust dose as needed

ADVERSE EFFECTS:
- Headache
- Dysmenorrhea
- Abdominal pain
- Pruritis

SPECIAL NURSING CONSIDERATIONS:
- Antibiotic activity greater than norfloxacin but
  equal to ciprofloxacin against gram-positive
  bacteria; slightly less effective than ciprofloxacin
  against gram-negative bacteria

- Drug well tolerated
- Superinfection by nonsusceptible organisms, e.g., fungi, may occur
- Drug ineffective against syphilis; serologic testing to exclude co-infection should be considered

PATIENT EDUCATION:
- Drink 2–3 L of fluid a day
- Take drug 2 hours apart from antacids
- Do not take drug with food
- Discontinue drug if rash, hives, rapid heartbeat, difficulty swallowing or breathing occur, and notify nurse or doctor immediately
- Avoid excessive sunlight; use sun protection factor (SPF 15) lotion when in the sun
- When used as second-line treatment for resistant TB, drug should be prescribed in consultation with a physician expert in the management of resistant TB

Ondansetron

BRAND NAME:
- Zofran

ACTION:
- Antiemetic; antagonizes serotonin receptors, thus preventing stimulation of vomiting center

INDICATIONS:
• Nausea and vomiting related to cancer chemotherapy

CONTRAINDICATIONS:
• Known hypersensitivity
• Use cautiously in hepatic failure, pregnancy,
nursing mothers

DOSAGE:
• IV:
—*Adults:* as single IV bolus dose of 32 mg 30
minutes prior to chemotherapy or
—Adults, children (≥ age 4): 0.15 mg/kg IV q 4
hours X 3, beginning 30 minutes prior to
chemotherapy
• Oral:
—*Adults (≥ 12 years):* 8 mg q 4 hours X 3
beginning 30 minutes before chemotherapy,
then q 8 hours X 1–2 days
—*Children (aged 4–12):* 4 mg tid
• Max dose 8 mg in hepatic failure

ADMINISTRATION:
• Oral, IV
• Administer IV dose as bolus, further diluted in
50 mL 5% dextrose or 0.9% sodium chloride
over 15 minutes
• DO NOT ADMINISTER with other drugs,
especially alkaline substances, as a precipitate
will form

DRUG INTERACTIONS:
- None significant

ADVERSE EFFECTS:
- Headache
- Constipation (11% when used in multiple-day treatment)
- *Uncommon:*
  - —Rash, weakness, xerostomia
  - —Transient increase in liver function tests
  - —Tachycardia
  - —Blurred vision

SPECIAL NURSING CONSIDERATIONS:
- 32 mg IVB single dose found superior to divided dosing
- As a rule, drug does not cause extrapyriamidal side effects since does not affect dopamine receptors (although rare isolated case has been reported)
- Breakthrough nausea and vomiting may occur approximately 19 hours after dose, especially with cisplatin chemotherapy, so need to provide continued antiemetic therapy
- Enhanced prevention of nausea/vomiting when combined with decadron
- Oral formulation indicated for moderately emetogenic chemotherapy

PATIENT EDUCATION:
- Increase oral fluids, dietary fiber to prevent constipation
- Report constipation
- Report headaches

Oxycodone Hydrochloride

BRAND NAMES:
- Roxicodone; Percocet (with acetaminophen), Percodan (with aspirin)

ACTION:
- Narcotic analgesic

INDICATIONS:
- Mild to moderately severe pain

CONTRAINDICATIONS:
- Known hypersensitivity to drug
- Use with caution in hepatic or renal dysfunction, hypothyroidism, Addison's disease, severe CNS depression, respiratory depression, head injury, elevated intracranial pressure, prostatic hypertrophy, urethral stricture

DOSAGE:
- Usual dose 5 mg q 6 hours
- More severe pain, tolerance:
  —10 mg PO q 4–6 hours
- Reduce dose in debilitated patients, or if receiving other CNS depressants

ADMINISTRATION:
- Oral
- Available as:
  —Roxicodone: 5 mg/mL, 20 mg/mL (Intensol), 5 mg tablets
  —Roxilox, Tylox, Roxicet 5/500 caplets: 5 mg oxycodone HCl and 500 mg acetaminophen
  —Oxycet, Percocet, Roxicet: 5 mg oxycodone HCl and 325 mg acetaminothen
  —Percodan, Codoxy, Roxiprin:
  > 4.5 mg oxycodone HCl
  > 0.38 mg oxycodone terephthalate
  > 325 mg aspirin

DRUG INTERACTIONS:
- Alcohol: increases CNS depression; AVOID concurrent use
- Anticoagulants, chemotherapy: aspirin-oxycodone combination may increase risk of bleeding; use acetaminophen—oxycodone preparation
- CNS depressants: additive CNS depressant effects; use together cautiously, if at all
- MAO inhibitors, tricyclic antidepressants: increases effect of both drugs

ADVERSE EFFECTS:
- Drowsiness, sedation, euphoria, mental clouding

- Respiratory depression, especially with overdosage
- Constipation
- Nausea, vomiting, dry mouth
- Psychologic and physical dependence
- Decreased libido

SPECIAL NURSING CONSIDERATIONS:
- Analgesic effect within 10–15 minutes after oral administration; max effect in 30–60 minutes; duration 3–6 hours
- Adverse effects milder than morphine
- Give smallest, effective dose to prevent development of tolerance and psychological dependence
- Assess bowel elimination status, with goal for bowel evacuation at least q 2 days

PATIENT EDUCATION:
- Avoid concurrent alcohol use
- Take only for pain, as addiction may occur
- Bowel regime including increased fluids, fiber in diet, exercise as tolerated, and stool softeners or cathartics
- Do not drive if feel dizzy or drowsy

Para-Aminosalicyclic Acid (PAS)

BRAND NAME:
- Tubasal

ACTION:
- Active against *Mycobacterium tuberculosis* only prevents synthesis of folic acid, causing cell death

INDICATIONS:
- Pulmonary tuberculosis, in conjunction with at least one other agent

CONTRAINDICATIONS:
- Known hypersensitivity
- Pregnancy
- Use with caution in patients with renal or hepatic dysfunction, gastric ulcer, congestive heart failure
- Use cautiously if at all in patients with G6PD deficiency, as may cause homolyric anemia

DOSAGE:
- *Adult:* 150 mg/kg (10–12 gin)in 2–4 equally divided doses q day
- *Children:* 150–300 mg/kg daily in 3–4 equally divided doses, not to exceed 10–12 gm/day

ADMINISTRATION:
- Oral, with meals to decrease GI distress or with aluminum hydroxide antacid

DRUG INTERACTIONS:
- Probenecid: inhibits renal excretion of PAS, thus potentially increasing toxicity; use together with caution
- Diphenhydrarnine: decrease GI absorption of PAS; avoid concurrent use
- Digoxin: may decrease digoxin absorption; monitor closely
- Warfarin: may increase hypoglycemic effects; monitor closely and adjust dose

ADVERSE EFFECTS:
- Nausea, vomiting, diarrhea, abdominal pain, anorexia
- Hypersensitivity (fever, rash, pruritis, vasculitis, joint pain, blood dyscrasias, hepatitis, jaundice)
- Loeffler's syndrome (high fever, leukocytosis, eosinophilia, cough, dyspnea, and pulmonary infiltrates)

SPECIAL NURSING CONSIDERATIONS:
- Drug is not first-line therapy
- Monitor patient for signs/symptoms of allergic reaction; discontinue all drugs if this occurs; drugs may be resumed one at a time to determine offending agent

- Monitor patient for signs/symptoms of Loeffler's syndrome: discontinue drug if these develop
- When used as second line for resistant TB, drug should be prescribed in consultation with a physician expert in management of resistant TB

PATIENT EDUCATION:
- Assess for and report high fever, cough, dyspnea immediately
- Discontinue drug if rash, itching, yellow skin develop; notify physician or nurse immediately
- Take with meals or aluminum-containing antacid if gastric distress develops

Paromomycin Sulfate

BRAND NAME:
- Humatin

ACTION:
- Broad-spectrum antibiotic agent

INDICATIONS:
- Treatment of intestinal amebiasis (acute and chronic), *Cryptosporidium, Entamoeba histolytica* (asymptomatic carrier)

CONTRAINDICATIONS:
- Prior hypersensitivity
- Intestinal obstruction

- Use with caution, *if at all,* in patients with ulcerative bowel lesions, as drug may then be absorbed systematically, causing renal toxicity

DOSAGE:
- *Adults and children:*
  —25 mg–35 mg/kg PO q d in 3 divided doses X 5–10 days

ADMINISTRATION:
- Available in 250 mg capsules
- Take *with meals*

DRUG INTERACTIONS:
- Drug is not absorbed systemically

ADVERSE EFFECTS:
- Skin rash Vertigo, headache
- At doses > 3 gm/day:
  —Nausea
  —Abdominal cramps
  —Diarrhea

SPECIAL NURSING CONSIDERATIONS:
- Drug is an aminoglycoside similar to neomycin
- Manage diarrhea symptoms of *Cryptosporidium* with Imodium, diphenoxylate, DTO, or octreotide (Sandostatin)

PATIENT EDUCATION:
- Drug administration
- Measures to decrease diarrhea
- Measures to prevent dehydration
- Perineal hygiene

Penicillin G Benzathine

BRAND NAMES:
- Bicillin, Megacillin

ACTION:
- Antibacterial agent; inhibits cell wall synthesis of microorganism

INDICATIONS:
- Syphilis

CONTRAINDICATIONS:
- Hypersensitivity to penicillin
- Use with caution if prior hypersensitivity to cephalosporins

DOSAGE:
- 2.4 million units IM X 1 (less than 1 year duration)
- 2.4 million units IM q week X 3 (> 1 year duration)

ADMINISTRATION:
- Deep IM into large muscle mass
- NEVER GIVE IV

Drug Profiles

DRUG INTERACTIONS:
- Probenecid: increases serum penicillin levels

ADVERSE EFFECTS:
- Hypersensitivity (rash, eosinophilia, urticaria, chills, fever, anaphylaxis)
- Discomfort and sterile abcesses at injection site
- Uncommon: blood dyscrasias, neuropathy, seizures

SPECIAL NURSING CONSIDERATIONS:
- Select injection site carefully: large muscle mass (e.g., gluteus maximus), and inject deeply

PATIENT EDUCATON:
- Safe sexual practices to avoid reinfection
- Report signs/symptoms of allergic reaction (rash, chills, fever, edema)

Penicillin G Potassium

BRAND NAME:
- Pfizerpen

ACTION:
- Antibacterial agent: inhibits cell wall synthesis of micro-organism

INDICATIONS:
- *S. pneumoniae* infections, other moderate to severe infections

CONTRAINDICATIONS:
- Hypersensitivity to penicillin
- Use with caution if hypersensitive to cephalosporin antibiotics

DOSAGE:
- Oral: 400,000–800,000 u q 6 hours
- IM/IV: 200,000–4 million q 4 hours
- May need to modify dose if renal impairment

ADMINISTRATION:
- Oral: administer at least 1 hour before or 2 hours after meals
- IM: reconstitute drug as directed. Give IM deep into large muscle mass
- IV: reconstitute as directed. Further dilute in 0.9% sodium chloride or 5% dextrose in water, and administer over 1–2 hours

DRUG INTERACTIONS:
- Aminoglycosides: synergism
- Rifampin: possible antagonism at high doses of penicillin
- Probenecid: increases serum level of penicillin. Use together as ordered

ADVERSE EFFECTS:
- Hypersensitivity reaction (rash, urticaria, chills, fever, anaphylaxis)
- Superinfection by nonsusceptible organisms (e.g., *Candida*)

- Thrombophlebitis
- Uncommon: neuropathy, hemolytic anemia, leukopenia, thrombocytopenia, exfoliative dermatitis
- Uncommon except at high doses: seizures, hyperkalemia

SPECIAL NURSING CONSIDERATIONS:
- Monitor for signs/symptoms of hypersensitivity during first and second doses
- Assess for signs/symptoms of bacterial or fungal superinfection

PATIENT EDUCATION:
- Report rash, fever. chills immediately
- Self-assessment for superinfections, such as oral *Candida*

Pentamidine Isethionate, Aerosolized

BRAND NAME:
- NebuPent (aerosolized pentamidine)

ACTION:
- Antiprotozoal agent

INDICATIONS:
- Prevention of *Pneumocystis carinii* pneumonia (PCP) in high-risk, HIV-infected patients with a past history of 1+ episodes of PCP, or a CD_4 lymphocyte count $\leq$ 200/mm^3

CONTRAINDICATIONS:
- Prior anaphylactic reaction to inhaled or parenteral pentamidine isethionate
- Use in pregnant or nursing females unless benefits outweigh risks

DOSAGE:
- 300 mg q 4 weeks by Respirgard II nebulizer
- 150 mg q month by Aerotech II 60 mg q 2 weeks by Fisoneb

ADMINISTRATION:
- Dissolve 1 vial (300 mg) by adding 3–6 mL sterile water for injection USP (not normal saline). Place in nebulizer resevoir
- Establish flow rate of 6–10 L/minute from a 40–50 PSI air or oxygen source, or air compressor (22–25 PSI)
- Deliver until nebulizer empty (15–30 minutes)

DRUG INTERACTIONS:
- DO NOT MIX drug solution with any other drugs
- DO NOT USE nebulizer to administer other drugs
- Normal saline: incompatible, forms precipitate

ADVERSE EFFECTS:
- Bronchospasm or cough
- With chronic use of aerosolized pentamidine, rarely:
  —Hypotension
  —Hypo- or hyperglycemia
  —Hypocalcemia
  —Anemia, thrombocytopenia, leukopenia
  —Hepatic or renal dysfunction
  —Pancreatitis
  —Stevens-Johnson syndrome
  —Ventricular tachycardia

SPECIAL NURSING CONSIDERATIONS:
- Drug may not be inhaled into lung apices if patient sitting, creating sanctuary
- Drug does not prophylaxe against extrapulmonary *Pneumocystis carinii*
- Patient may still develop acute PCP so any symptom of pulmonary infection (dyspnea, fever, cough) must be evaluated promptly
- CXR and clinical presenstation of PCP may be atypical after receiving nebupent
- Bronchospasm or cough may occur, especially in patients with history of smoking or asthma. May require inhaled bronchodilator prior to pentamidine
- Drug can be administered at home if support personnel available) or in clinic

- Must rule out tuberculosis if drug administered in clinic. Use measures to minimize exposure of drug to health care workers. Drug should be administered in individual rooms or booths with negative pressure ventilation and exhausted to outside. Health care workers should wear particulate respirators when in room. If coughing, keep patient in room until cough disappears
- Efficiency (delivery of drug to lungs) 21% with Aerotech II, 5% Respirgard II, and 16% Fisoneb (Sinaidone et al, 1991)
- Refer to home care agency skilled in aerosolized pentamidine administration for home therapy

PATIENT EDUCATION:
- Report signs/symptoms of pulmonary infection
- Drug administration technique

Pentamidine Isethionate, Parenteral

BRAND NAME:
- Pentam 300

ACTION:
- Antiprotozoal agent

INDICATIONS:
- Treatment of pneumonia caused by *Pneumocystis carlnil* (PCP)

CONTRAINDICATIONS:
- Use with caution in patients with hypertension, hypotension, hypoglycemia, hyperglycemia, hypocalcemia, leukopenia, anemia, thrombocytopenia, and renal or hepatic dysfunction

DOSAGE:
- *Adults and children:* 4 mg/kg IV or IM q d X 14 days

ADMINISTRATION:
- Dissolve 300 mg vial contents with 3 mL sterile water for injection (USP)
- Withdraw ordered dose and administer IM, or after diluted with 3–5 mL, further dilute ordered dose in 50–250 mL D5W and administer over 60 minutes

DRUG INTERACTIONS:
- Didanosine: increased risk of pancreatitis; hold didanosine during pentamidine therapy
- Foscarnet: may develop severe hypocalcemia, increased risk of nephrotoxicity; AVOID combination if possible; hydrate well
- Zalcitabine: increased risk of pancreatitis; hold zalcitabine during pentamidine therapy

ADVERSE EFFECTS:
- Hypotension with rapid IV administration, Bess commonly after IM
- Rash

- Nausea, vomiting
- Nephrotoxicity
- Cardiac arrhythmias
- Neutropenia (15% of patients), thrombocytopenia
- Pancreatitis
- Hypocalcemia
- Hypoglycemia, then hyperglycemia
- Sterile abcesses after IM injection

SPECIAL NURSING CONSIDERATIONS:
- Monitor BP closely during and after drug administration
- Monitor baseline BUN, serum creatinine, glucose, liver function studies, serum calcium, and EKG and periodically during treatment
- Cure rate 60–80% if receive full course of therapy

PATIENT EDUCATI ON:
- Signs/symptoms of hypo-, hyperglycemia and to report them immediately
- To report any changes in condition

Pentoxifylline

BRAND NAME:
- Trentyl

ACTION:
- Tri-substituted xanthine, appears to inhibit tumor necrosis factor (TNF), which accompanies progressive HIV infection and wasting syndrome

INDICATIONS:
- U.S. Food and Drug Administration approved for claudication
- Investigational use to prevent AIDS-related cachexia (wasting syndrome)

CONTRAINDICATIONS:
- Per protocol
- Patients intolerant to caffeine, theophylline, theobromine (methylxanthines)

DOSAGE:
- 400 mg PO tid

ADMINISTRATION:
- Oral; available as 400 mg extended-release tablets. Take with meals

DRUG INTERACTIONS:
- Antihypertensives: increases hypotensive effect; monitor blood pressure closely and modify dose as needed
- Warfarin: increases anticoagulation: AVOID if possible or modify warfarin dose

ADVERSE EFFECTS:
- Headache, dizziness, CNS disturbances (mild)
- Nausea, vomiting, dyspepsia (occasionally)

SPECIAL NURSING CONSIDERATIONS:
- Patient may show increase in CD_4 counts
- Shows promise in reversing weight loss, promoting weight gain, and improving general sense of well-being
- U.S. Food and Drug Administration-approved in the treatment of claudication to improve blood flow in capillaries by making erythrocytes more flexible and decreasing blood viscosity

PATIENT EDUCATION:
- Self-administration of drug per protocol
- Notify nurse or physician if side effects develop

Permethrin

BRAND NAME:
- Elimite 5% cream

ACTION:
- Topical scabicide agent

INDICATIONS:
- Treatment of scabies infestation *(Sarcoptes scalieli*

CONTRAINDICATIONS:
- Known hypersensitivity
- Use in pregnancy, unless benefit outweighs risk
- Use in nursing mothers, unless benefit outweighs risk

DOSAGE:
- *Adults and children (> 2 months):* one dose: thoroughly rub cream into skin starting from head to soles of feet. Infants should have treatment of scalp, forehead, temple. One dose is curative

ADMINISTRATION:
- Leave cream on 8–14 hours, then wash off with water (shower or bah)

DRUG INTERACTIONS:
- None

ADVERSE EFFECTS:
- Mild, transient burning and stinging after application (10%)
- Pruritis (7%)
- Erythema, numbness, tingling, rash (1–2%)

SPECIAL NURSING CONSIDERATIONS:
- Avoid contact with eyes
- Itching, mild stinging, or burning may occur after application
- Temporary itching may occur up to 2 weeks after application, resolving after 4 weeks.

PATIENT EDUCATION:
- If itching persists, report to physician or nurse

Perphenazine

BRAND NAME:
- Trilafon

ACTION:
- Antipsychotic agent used as an antiemetic agent
- Blocks dopamine receptors in chemoreceptor trigger zone

INDICATIONS:
Management of psychotic disorders
- Used as an antiemetic based on clinical efficacy

CONTRAINDICATIONS:
- Hypertension
- Nursing mothers
- Blood dyscrasias
- Sulfite sensitivity (when given IM)
- Coma

DOSAGE:
- Oral: 4 mg q 4–6 hours
- IM/IV: 3–5 mg IV bolus q 4–6 hours or 3–5 mg IV bolus then infusion at 1 mg/hour X 10 hours

ADMINISTRATION:
- Oral
- IM or IV bolus

DRUG INTERACTIONS:
- Antidepressants: increase parkinsonian symptoms; use together cautiously
- Barbiturates, other CNS depressants: increase CNS depression; use together cautiously

ADVERSE EFFECTS:
- Extrapyramidal reactions:
    - —Opisthotonus
    - —Trismus
    - —Torticollis
    - —Motor restlessness
    - —Oculogyric crises
    - —Dystonia
    - —Tongue protrusion
- Sedation
- Dry mouth, mild photosensitivity

SPECIAL NURSING CONSIDERATIONS:
- Injection contains sodium bisulfite: do not administer to patients allergic to sulfltes; use cautiously in patients with asthma

- Benadryl 50 mg IM or IV rapidly reverses extrapyramidal reactions
- Usually, maximum dose in 24 hour period is 30 mg for hospitalizod patients, and 15 mg for outpatients

PATIENT EDUCATION:
- Report signs/symptoms of extrapyramidal side effects imediately
- Self administration of oral Trilafon to prevent nausea/vomiting
- Notify physician or nurse if nausea/vomiting is unrelieved by drug

Phenytoin Sodium

BRAND NAME:
- Dilantin

ACTION:
- Anticonvulsant; inhibits seizure activity in motor cortex

INDICATIONS:
- Control of tonic-clonic and psychomotor seizures; prevention of seizures during or after neurosurgery

CONTRAINDICATIONS:
- Hypersensitivity to drug
- Use with caution in persons with porphyria, pregnancy, or in renal or hepatic dysfunction

DOSAGE:
- *Adults:* if loading dose ordered: 1 gm IV given at 50 mg/min, or orally in 3 divided doses; maintenance: 300 mg PO q d (extended) or 100 mg tid (extended or prompt)
- *Children:* maintenance 4–8 mg/kg; children > 6 years old may need max 300 mg/day

ADMINISTRATION:
- IV push: not to exceed 50 mg/min; do not mix in solution; give IVP via 0.9% normal saline mainline IV
- Oral: prompt or extended kapseals

DRUG INTERACTIONS:
- Acute alcohol ingestion: increases serum phenytoin levels
- Chronic alcohol ingestion: decreases serum phenytoin levels
- Chloramphenicol, diazepam, dicumarol, H_2antagonists, isoniazid, phenothiazides, salicylates, sulfonamides: increases phenytoin Iserum levels
- Carbamazepine, sucralfate, calcium-containing antacids: decreases phenytoin levels

- Phenobarbital, valproic acid, sodium valproate: may increase or decrease phenytoin levels
- Corticosteroids, coumarin anticoagulants, doxycycline, oral contraceptives, furosemide, rifampin, theophylline: decreases efficacy of each of these drugs when given concurrently with phenytoin

ADVERSE EFFECTS:
- Rash (measles-like); rare exfoliative dermatitis, Stevens-Johnson syndrome
- Nausea, vomiting
- Gingival hyperplasia
- nystagmus, confusion, ataxia, slurred speech (dose-related)
- Blood dyscrasias (uncommon)
- Toxic hepatitis (uncommon)
- Hypersensitivity syndrome (arthralgias, eosinophilia, fever, rash, liver dysfunction)

SPECIAL NURSING CONSIDERATIONS:
- Abrupt withdrawal in epileptic patients may precipitate status epilepticus
- Discontinue if skin rash develops to prevent development of Stevens-Johnson syndrome
- Drug has reportedly been related to development of lymphadenopathy in some patients
- Therapeutic range (serum) 10–20 µg/mL
- Assess serum phenytoin level if CNS symptoms develop

PATIENT EDUCATION:
- Avoid alcoholic beverages
- Take medication as prescribed
- Notify doctor or nurse if unable to take drug
- Stop drug and call doctor or nurse if skin rash develops
- Use regular oral hygiene and gum care to prevent gingival hyperplasia

Podofilox

BRAND NAME:
- Condylox

ACTION:
- Keratolytic agent

INDICATIONS:
- Exophytic genital warts *(Condyloma acuminatum*

CONTRAINDICATIONS:
- Perianal or mucosal membrane warts
- Known hypersensitivity

DOSAGE:
- Topical solution 0.5%
- Apply to affected lesion(s) once every 12 hours X 3 days; wait 4 days; repeat same cycle up to 4 cycles until warts disappear

ADMINISTRATION:
- Apply with cotton-tipped applicator that comes with medication directly to wart
- Use least amount of solution to cover the wart
- Never use more than 0.5 mL/day or apply to > 10 cm^2 (4 inches) of wart
- Allow area to dry well before releasing skin (skin stabilized by fingers)

DRUG INTERACTIONS:
- None; topical application

ADVERSE EFFECTS:
- Local burning and pain
- Less than 5% of patients:
    —Painful intercourse
    —Vesicle formation
    —Tingling
    —Crusting, peeling
    —Bleeding
    —Erosion
- Systemic (if exceed directed use): insomnia, dizziness, vomiting, hematuria

SPECIAL NURSING CONSIDERATIONS:
- Avoid contact with eyes
- If lesion has not disappeared after 4 weeks, consider alternative therapy (e.g., cryosurgery)
- Additional applications DO NOT improve efficacy but do increase risk of systemic absorption and toxicity

PATIENT EDUCATION:
- Drug is for external use only
- Avoid contact with eyes; if this occurs, wash copiously with water and see physician or ophthalmologist
- Patient Information leaflet should be obtained when prescription is filled
- Demonstrate procedure and identify lesion(s) to be treated

Podophyllum Resin 25% in Tincture of Benzoin

BRAND NAMES:
- Pod-ben 25, Podoben, Podolin

ACTION:
- Keratolytic agent; caustic action destroying warts

INDICATIONS:
- Human papilloma virus (HPV)-induced genital wads *(Condylorna acurninaturn)*

CONTRAINDICATIONS:
- Known hypersensitivity
- Cervical, intraurethral, or oral warts
- Pregnant women

DOSAGE:
- Treatment with 10–25% solution, limited to area < 10 cm^2, with total volume < 0.5 mL per session. Vaginal warts limited to area < 2 cm^2

ADMINISTRATION:
- Apply topically, one drop at a time to prevent contact with normal tissue. Wash off after 1–4 hours using soap and water (all drug must be washed off). Apply weekly to q 10 days X 4
- Protect skin adjacent to treatment site by applying petroleum or flexible collodion
- When treating vaginal warts, treated area must be dry before removing speculum
- Lesions become necrotic in 24–48 hours, begin to slough off slowly in 72 hours. and gradually disappear without scarring

DRUG INTERACTIONS:
- None

ADVERSE EFFECTS:
- Usually dependent on duration of drug application, increasing if left on > 4 hours
- CNS side effects: altered sensorium, hallucinations, ataxia
- Peripheral neuropathy, occurring 2 weeks after application, may progressively worsen up to 3 months, lasting up to 9 months

- Other systemic side effects if absorbed: nausea, vomiting, abdominal pain, diarrhea, bone marrow depression, hepatotoxicity, renal failure

SPECIAL NURSING CONSIDERATIONS:
- Applied by physician or trained nurse ONLY
- Does not cure HPV infection, rather, removes exophytic warts and improves symptoms of infection
- Alternative therapy to cryotherapy
- Mucosal warts most likely to respond; cryotherapy should be used for vaginal or cervical wads by an experienced gynecologist
- Resin no longer recommended for treatment of anal warts because of possible damage to normal mucosa
- AVOID contact with eyes, mucosal membranes as very irritating
- AVOID applying to large areas, using excessive amounts, allowing to remain on mucosa for > 4 hours, or application to recently biopsied areas as systemic absorption may occur
- Patients with atypical, pigmented, or persistent wads should have the lesions biopsied to rule out malignancy
- Papanicolaou test (Pap smear) should be done annually on all women with anogenital warts

PATIENT EDUCATION:
- Report signs/symptoms of systemic absorption: change in mental status, peripheral neuropathy, any change in condition
- Application is painful in affected area, but will resolve in a short time

Prednisone

BRAND NAME:
- Deltasone

ACTION:
- Corticosteroid

INDICATIONS:
- Treatment may be prescribed as an adjunct to other anti-infectives for the treatment of moderately severe *Pneumocystis carinii* pneumonia ($pO_2 < 70$ mm Hg)in patients able to take oral medications

CONTRAINDICATIONS:
- Known hypersensitivity Systemic fungal infections

DOSAGE:
- *Adults and children > 13 years old:* 40 mg bid X 5 days; 40 mg q d X 5 days; 20 mg q d X 11 days

ADMINISTRATION:
- Oral, with meals or food

DRUG INTERACTIONS:
- Amphoterian B, potassium-depleting diuretics: increased potassium loss
- Coumadin: decreased effect; may need to increase dose
- Oral contraceptives: may inhibit steroid metabolism

ADVERSE EFFECTS:
- CNS toxicity (headache, vertigo)
- Hyperglycemia
- Thrush
- Menstrual irregularities
- Herpes simplex superinfection
- Peptic ulcer, gastritis
- Tuberculosis
- Sodium and fluid retention
- Opportunistic infections
- Petechiae and ecchymosis
- Adrenal insufficiency

SPECIAL NURSING CONSIDERATIONS:
- Prednisone should begin within 24–72 hours of initial anti-infective therapy
- Recommendation for adjunctive therapy based on limited data; may be variation in usage

- Take prednisone with food or milk
- Follow taper schedule as directed
- Report any abdominal pain, bleeding, or any change in general condition

Primaquine Phosphate

BRAND NAME:
- Primaquine Phosphate tablets

ACTION:
- Antimalarial agent
- Antiprotozoal agent

INDICATIONS:
- Malaria prophylaxis
- Second-line therapy in combination with clindamycin for management of *Pneumonocystiscarinii* pneumonia in patients not acutely ill ($pO_2 > 60$ mm Hg) useful for patients allergic to sulfonamides

CONTRAINDICATIONS:
- Acutely ill patients with risk to develop granulocytopenia (e.g., rheumatoid arthritis)
- Patients receiving other hemolytic or myeloid bone marrow suppressive therapy
- Pregnant or nursing women

DOSAGE:
- Primaquin 15 mg (base) PO q d and Clindamycin 600 mg IV q 6 hours or Clindamycin 300–450 mg PO q 6 hours X 21 days

ADMINISTRATION:
- Oral X 21 days
- Take with meals to decrease GI upset

DRUG INTERACTIONS:
- Quinacrine: potentiates toxicity; avoid concurrent use, or use if patient recently received quinacrine

ADVERSE EFFECTS:
- Acute hemolysis (hemolytic anemia) may occur to patients with G6PD deficiency
- Nausea, vomiting, epigastric distress
- Mild-moderate abdominal cramping
- Headache
- Pruritis
- Decrease in visual accommodation

SPECIAL NURSING CONSIDERATIONS/ PATIENT EDUCATION:
- Patients ar risk for G6PD deficiency should be screened before drug is given (black males, men of Mediterranean descent, from India, or from Far East)

- Some patients may receive concurrent corticosteroids
- Teach patient
  —To continue full 21-day regime even if feeling better
  —To report any change in condition
  —To report any darkening of urine

Probenecid

BRAND NAME:
- Benemid

ACTION:
- Increases renal excretion of uric acid by preventing tubular reabsorption
- Inhibits renal tubular secretion of penicillins and cephalosporins, thus increasing antibiotic serum levels

INDICATIONS:
- Gouty arthritis, gout-related hyperuricemia; adjunct to antibiotic therapy

CONTRAINDICATIONS:
- Hypersensitivity to drug
- Children < 2 years old
- Blood dyscrasias, uric acid-induced kidney stones
- Use cautiously in renal dysfunction

DOSAGE:
- Adjunct to penicillin or cephalosporin
  —*Adult, children > 50 kg:* 500 mg PO qid
  —*Children < 50 kg or ages 2–14:* 25 mg/kg PO,
  then 10 mg/kg qid
- Hyperuricemia/gout: (after gouty attack over):
  250 mg bid X 1 week, then 500 mg bid-max
  1 gm bid; maintenance: 500 mg q d X 6 months
- Available as 500 mg tablets

ADMINISTRATION:
- Oral, with food or milk if gastric distress

DRUG INTERACTIONS:
- Salicylates: prevents uric acid excretion; do not
  use together
- Oral hypoglycemics: enhances action; monitor
  for hypoglycemia
- Indocin, acetaminophen, naproxyn, lorazepam,
  rifampin: increases serum levels; monitor for
  toxicity and dose-reduce

ADVERSE EFFECTS:
- Headache
- Hypotension, dizziness
- Nausea/vomiting, anorexia
- Pruritis, alopecia, flushing
- Fever

SPECIAL NURSING CONSIDERATIONS:
- Single-dose treatment of gonorrhea
—Adults: 3.5 gm ampicillin plus 1 gm
probenecid PO or 1 gm probenecid PO 30
minutes prior to 4.8 million units of aqueous
penicillin G procaine IM in 2 injections
- Monitor renal function (BUN, creatinine) during
chronic therapy

PATIENT EDUCATION:
- Increase fluids to 2–3 L/day
- Take medication as prescribed
- Avoid aspirin

Prochlorperazine

BRAND NAME:
- Compazine

ACTION:
- Antiemetic agent; blocks dopamine receptors in
chemotherapy trigger zone and decreases
vagal stimulation of vomiting center

INDICATIONS:
- Severe nausea/vomiting

CONTRAINDICATIONS:
- Known hypersensitivity
- Comatose states
- In presence of large amounts of CNS depres-
sants (e.g., alcohol)

DOSAGE:
- Dose adjusted to response of individual: may require > 40 mg/day
- *Adult:* 5–10 mg PO qid (usual max 40 mg/day); 2.5–10 mg IV up to qid (usual max 40 mg/day); 25 mg bid rectal suppository

ADMINISTRATION:
- Oral: immediate (5 or 10 mg tablets) or spansules (10, 15, 30 mg)
- IM
- IV: adminster IVP or IVB slowly, at least 5 mg/minute
- Rectal: suppository

DRUG INTERACTIONS:
- Antacids: decrease oral prochlorperazine absorption; separate by 2 hours
- Antidepressants: increase parkinsonian symptoms; use together cautiously
- Barbiturates: decreases prochlorperazine effect; may need to increase dose

ADVERSE EFFECTS:
- Extrapyrimidal side effects (tongue protrusion, trismus, akathesia, tremor, insomnia)
- Sedation
- Orthostatic hypotension
- Blurred vision
- Dry mouth, constipation
- Rash, urticaria
- Rarely, exfoliative dermatitis

SPECIAL NURSING CONSIDERATIONS:
- Extrapyramidal side effects (EPS) rapidly reversed by diphenhydramine 50 mg IV. Can give 25 mg IV prior to large IV doses of prochlorperazine to prevent EPS
- Dose adjusted to patient response; higher doses may be used as antiemetic prior to chemotherapy

PATIENT EDUCATION:
- Avoid using machinery or driving a car when feel drowsy
- Self-medication to prevent nausea/vomiting
- Report rash, bothersome side effects
- Change position slowly

Pyrantel Pamoate

BRAND NAME:
- Antiminth

ACTION:
- Antihelminthic agent

INDICATIONS:
- Use in the eradication of *Enterobius vermicularis* (pinworm), *Ascaris lumbricoides* (roundworm), *Ancylostoma duodenale* (hookworm), *Necator americanus* (hookworm) and *Trichostrongylus orientalis* (hairworm)

- Alternative treatment for *Strongyloides stercoralis*

CONTRAINDICATIONS:
- Known hypersensitivity to drug
- Use with caution in patients with hepatic dysfunction

DOSAGE:
- *Adults and children > 2 years old:*
  —Ascariasis, enterobiasis, trichostrongyliasis, or hookworm: 11 mg/kg (pyrantel) given as a single dose (max 1 gm)
  —Patients with enterobiasis (pinworm) should repeat dose in 2 weeks
  —*Strongyloides stercoralis:* repeat q 2 weeks X 2

ADMINISTRATION:
- Oral suspension, 250 mg (pyrantel) per 5 mL
- Mix with milk or juice

DRUG INTERACTIONS:
- Piperazine: antagonism; do not use concurrently

ADVERSE EFFECTS:
- Mild, infrequent, transient
- Nausea, vomiting, tenesmus, anorexia, diarrhea
- Abdominal cramping
- Headache, dizziness, drowsiness
- Rash, fever, weakness
- Transient increased liver function tests

SPECIAL NURSING CONSIDERATIONS:
- Drug action
- Hygienic measures to prevent reinfection

PATIENT EDUCATION:
- Alert nurse or physician if abdominal cramps, nausea, vomiting persist

Pyrazinamide (PZA)

BRAND NAME:
- Pyrazinamide tablets

ACTION:
- Antituberculin agent

INDICATIONS:
- Initial treatment of active TB in adults and children in combination with other agents, (e.g., isoniazid, and rifampin)

CONTRAINDICATIONS:
- Severe hepatic damage
- Known hypersensitivity
- Acute gout
- Pregnant or nursing women unless benefit outweighs risk

DOSAGE:
- *Adults and children:*
  —15–30 mg/kg q d (max 2–3 gm) for first 2 months of 6+ month regime or can be given in a dose of 50–70 mg/kg 2 X/week. Isoniazid and rifampin, or other antituberculin drugs would be continued for the full regime

ADMINISTRATION:
- Available in 500 mg tablets

DRUG INTERACTIONS:
- None known

ADVERSE EFFECTS:
- Fever, porphyria, dysuria
- Hepatotoxicity (dose-related)
- Nausea, vomiting, anorexia
- Thrombocytopenia, sideroblastic anemia (rare)
- Mild arthralgias, myalgias
- Rash, pruritis

SPECIAL NURSING CONSIDERATIONS/ PATIENT EDUCATION:
- Patients with diabetes mellitus should be monitored closely
- Drug should be discontinued if gouty arthritis develops
- Teach patient to notify doctor or nurse if fever, loss of appetite, malaise, nausea, vomiting, dark urine, jaundice, pain, or swelling of joints occurs. Need to complete FULL course of treatment, without missing doses

Pyrethrins

BRAND NAME:
- RID lice-killing shampoo

ACTION:
- Pediculicide that kills head, body, pubic lice, and their eggs

INDICATIONS:
- Head lice *(Pediculus humanus capitis)*
- Body lice *(Pediculus humanus humanus)*
- Pubic or crab lice *(Phthirus pubis)*

CONTRAINDICATIONS:
- Use with caution in ragweed-sensitized patients

DOSAGE:
- Available in 2, 4, 8 fluid oz. bottles. Do not exceed 2 applications within 24 hours

ADMINISTRATION:
- Shake well; apply undiluted to dry hair, scalp, infested body areas EXCEPT EYELASHES AND EYEBROWS until area wet. Leave on 10 MINUTES, then wash well with warm water and soap or shampoo. Comb area with nit comb to remove dead lice and eggs. Repeat treatment in 7–10 days to eradicate newly hatched lice

DRUG INTERACTIONS:
- Drug rinses away after treatment
- Active drug ingredients poorly absorbed through skin

ADVERSE EFFECTS:
- Drug to be used EXTERNALLY ONLY

SPECIAL NURSING CONSIDERATIONS:
- Consult dermatologist for treatment of infestation of eyebrows or eyelashes

PATIENT EDUCATION:
- Teach self-administration, avoiding swallowing, inhalation, or contact with eyes or mucous membranes
- Do not use near food
- Do not reuse empty container
- Discard by wrapping in 2+ thicknesses of newspapers, then place in plastic bag and discard

Pyridoxine Hydrochloride

BRAND NAMES:
- Beesix, Hexa-Betalin, Rodex

ACTION:
- Vitamin B_6 is a water-soluble vitamin
- Prevents vitamin deficiency, anemia, neuritis in patients taking isoniazid

INDICATIONS:
• Mycobacteria treated with isoniazid

CONTRAINDICATIONS:
• Known hypersensitivity
• Patients taking levodopa

DOSAGE:
• May give 100 mg PO q d X 3 weeks, then
  —25 mg PO q d X 12 months
  —If patient receiving didanosine (ddl), may give
  50 mg q d X 12 months

ADMINISTRATION:
• Oral

DRUG INTERACTIONS:
Levodopa: decrease levodopa effect; avoid
  concomitant use
• Phenobarbital: decrease phenobarbital level;
  may need to increase dose or avoid concurrent
  use
• Phenytoin: may decrease phenytoin level; may
  need to increase dose or avoid concurrent use

ADVERSE EFFECTS:
• *Uncommon:*
  —Nausea
  —Headache
  —Paresthesia
  —Somnolence
  —Increased SGOT

SPECIAL NURSING CONSIDERATIONS:
• Monitor liver function studies baseline and periodically

PATIENT EDUCATION:
• Take as directed
• Importance of compliance with long-term regimen
• Report signs/symptoms of side effects

Pyrimethamine

BRAND NAME:
• Daraprin (pyrimethamine 25 mg)

ACTION:
• Antiparasite

INDICATIONS:
• Chemoprophylaxis of malaria (low doses)
• Treatment of *Toxoplasmosis gondii*

CONTRAINDICATIONS:
• Known hypersensitivity
• Patients with megaloblastic anemia due to folate deficiency
• Use with caution in patients with renal or hepatic dysfunction
• Use with caution, if at all, in pregnant or nursing mothers

DOSAGE:
* Toxoplasmosis
  —*Children:* 1 mg/kg divided into 2 doses;
  decrease dose to 50% 2–4 days later and
  continue X 1 month. Combine with pediatric
  dose of sulfonamide
  —*Adult:* acute infection: 100–200 mg loading
  dose, then 50–100 mg/day PO X 6 weeks
  PLUS sulfadiazine 200 mg/kg or
  trisulfapyrimidine 4–8 gm/day POX at least 6
  weeks (may be dosereduced if drug toxicity)
  —*Adult:* suppressive therapy: pyrimethamine
  25–50 mg 2 X/week to q d plus sulfadiazine (75
  mg/kg) or trisulfapyrimidine 2–4 gm/day PO
  2 X/week–q d, indefinitely

ADMINISTRATION:
* Orally, give with meals if nausea develops

DRUG INTERACTIONS:
* Sulfadiazine: synergism; equal synergism with
  sulfamethazine, and sulfamerazine
* Lorazepam: may increase hepatotoxicity; use
  together cautiously

ADVERSE EFFECTS:
* Hypersensitivity reactions
* Anorexia, vomiting
* Megaloblastic anemia, leukopenia,
  thrombocytopenia, pancytopenia

- Atrophic glossitis
- Hematuria
- Cardiac rhythm disturbances

SPECIAL NURSING CONSIDERATIONS:
- Baseline CBC, platelets, and semiweekly blood counts should be monitored
- Dosage of pyrimethamine used to treat toxoplasmosis is 10–20 X antimalaria dose; value of folinic acid to protect the bone marrow has not been demonstrated in controlled clinical studies
- > 90% of patients will respond clinically by 14 days; if symptoms persist, brain biopsy indicated (toxoplasmosis with brain lesion)
- If allergic to sulfa drugs, alternative regimen is pyrimethamine 200 mg loading dose then 100 mg PO q d PLUS clindamycin 450 mg tid (or 600 mg IV q 6 hours) X 3–6 weeks
- If nausea persists, discuss dose reduction with physician

PATIENT EDUCATION:
- Assess for skin rash, stop drug if rash develops, and notify nurse or doctor immediately
- Report any changes in condition, especially sore throat, pallor, purpura, glossitis, blood in urine
- Keep medication out of reach of children

Quinacrine Hydrochloride

BRAND NAME:
- Atabrine

ACTION:
- Antiparasitic agent

INDICATIONS:
Giardiasis; cestodiasis (tapeworms); suppression
of malaria

CONTRAINDICATIONS:
- Known hypersensitivity
- Pregnancy
- Concomitant use with primaquine
- Use cautiously in patients with hepatic, renal
cardiac disease; alcoholism, porphyria, G6PD
deficiency; psoriasis

DOSAGE:
- Giardiasis:
  —*Adult:* 100 mg PO tid X 5–7 days
  —*Children:* 7 mg/kg/day in 3 divided doses
  (max 300 mg/day) after meals, X 5 days
- Tapeworms:
  —Bland, nonfat diet then fasting night before
  treatment
  —*Adults:* 200 mg PO q 10 minutes X 4 plus
  sodium bicarbonate; 600 mg PO with each dose
  (to reduce nausea and vomiting)

—*Children age 11–14 years:* 150–200 mg PO q 10 min X 4 (total dose 600 mg) with sodium bicarbonate 300 mg with each dose
—*Children age 5–10 years:* total dose 400 mg
—Saline purge 1–2 hours later
• Malaria:
—*Adults, children > 8 years old:* 200 mg PO with 1 gm sodium bicarbonate q 6 hours X 5 doses, then 100 mg tid X 6 days (total dose 2.8 gm in 7 days)

ADMINISTRATION:
• Administer after meals, with a full glass of water or fruit juice
• Tablet is bitter if crushed; disguise in honey or jam for children
• Available in 100 mg tablets

DRUG INTERACTIONS:
• Primaquine: increases primaquine toxicity; NEVER give together
• Hepatotoxic drugs: increases hepatotoxic damage; monitor liver function tests closely, avoid concurrent use if possible

ADVERSE EFFECTS:
• Headache
• Dizziness
• Anorexia, nausea, diarrhea
• Rarely, vomiting
• Skin eruptions, rarely exfoliative dermatitis
• With prolonged use, rare aplastic anemia

SPECIAL NURSING CONSIDERATIONS:
- Drug can be fatal if overdosed; if overdose suspected, induce emesis or gastric layage. Signs/symptoms of overdosage: CNS excitement (restlessness, insomnia, psychic stimulation, convulsions, nausea, vomiting, diarrhea, cramps)
- Patients on prolonged therapy should receive periodic ophthalmologic exams to identify reversible corneal edema
- Drug is concentrated in liver

PATIENT EDUCATION:
- Keep drug out of reach of children
- Yellow color of urine and skin is due to medication and is temporary
- Report any visual disturbances (e.g., haloes around light, blurred vision, difficulty focusing) immediately

Rifabutin (Ansamycin)

BRAND NAME:
- Mycobutin

ACTION:
- Antimycobacterial agent

INDICATIONS:
- Prevention of disseminated *Mycobacterium avium* complex (MAC) in patients with advanced HIV infection

CONTRAINDICATIONS:
- Known hypersensitivity reaction to rifabutin or other rifamycins
- Patients with active tuberculosis
- Use when risks outweigh benefits in pregnant (first trimester), or breast-feeding women

DOSAGE:
- 150 mg bid

ADMINISTRATION:
- Oral; may divide dose and/or give with food if nausea occurs

DRUG INTERACTIONS:
- Zidovudine (AZT): decreases serum drug levels of AZT but does not affect AZT inhibition of HIV
- Anticoagulants, corticosteroids, cyclosporine, dapsone, digoxin, oral contraceptives, oral hypoglycemics, quinidine: rifabutin may decrease drug effect and dose may need to be increased
- Anticonvulsants, barbiturates. beta-antagonists, diazepam, ketoconazole, diazepam, theophylline, verapamil: drug effect may be decreased when given concurrently with rifabutin, and may need to increase dose

ADVERSE EFFECTS:
- Neutropenia; less commonly, thrombocytopenia. anemia
- Increased SGOT, SGPT
- Discolored urine
- Rash
- Nausea, vomiting, diarrhea, abdominal pain, taste perversion
- Headache
- Myalgia, arthralgia

SPECIAL NURSING CONSIDERATIONS:
- Do not give drug to patients with active TB as patient may develop strain resistant to rifabutin and to rifampin
- Monitor LFTs if patient has severe liver dysfunction or is receiving hepatotoxic drugs
- Monitor white blood count, absolute neutrophil count, at least initially, while taking the drug

PATIENT EDUCATION:
- Signs/symptoms of MAC, as well as tuberculosis, and to report these immediately
- Signs/symptoms of myositis (muscle weakness with myalgias) or uveitis (red eye) and to report this immediately

- Possible brown-orange discoloration of urine, feces, sputum, perspiration, tears, skin may occur; also, soft contact lens may be permanently stained
- Women should avoid hormonal contraceptives

Rifampin

BRAND NAME:
- Rifadin

ACTION:
- Antimycobacterial agent inhibiting bacterial RNA synthesis

INDICATIONS:
- All forms of tuberculosis, in conjunction with at least one other antituberculin agent; also, treatment of asymptomatic carriers of *N. meningitidis*

CONTRAINDICATIONS:
- Known hypersensitivity
- Use cautiously in patients with liver dysfunction
- Pregnancy, nursing mothers: use only if benefits outweigh risks

DOSAGE:
- M. tuberculosis:
  —*Adults:* 600 mg PO q d or IV if unable to take oral X 6–9 months
  —*Children > 5 years:* 10–20 mg/kg PO (max 300 mg) q d

ADMINISTRATION:
- Available as 150 mg and 300 mg capsules; IV vial of 600 mg
- Administer 1 hour before or 2 hours after meals

DRUG INTERACTIONS:
- Alcohol, hepatotoxic medications: increase risk of hepatotoxicity; avoid concurrent use
- Para-aminosalicylate sodium: decrease absorption of rifampin; give 8–12 hours apart
- Probecnecid: may decrease rifampin levels; increase dose as needed
- Oral contraceptives: decreases effectiveness; use alternative contraception
- Ketoconazole, fluconazole: decreases effectiveness of both drugs; may need to increase doses
- Oral hypoglycemics, anticoagulants, corticosterolds, dapsone, anticonvulsants: decreases effectiveness of these drugs; doses may need to be increased

ADVERSE EFFECTS:
- Drowsiness
- Transient abnormalities in liver function tests
- Flu-like syndrome

Drug Profiles

- Discoloration (red-orange) of body fluids
- *Less common:*
  - —Blood dyscrasias
  - —Pruritis, rash
  - —Nausea, vomiting, abdominal pain
  - —Headache, fatigue, confusion

SPECIAL NURSING CONSIDERATIONS:
- Monitor all patients baseline, periodically: CBC, liver function, renal function
- Monitor patients with liver dysfunction very closely; monitor SGPT (serum glutamic pyruvic transaminase) and SGOT (serum glutamic oxaloacetic transaminase) baseline and q 2–4 weeks during therapy. Discontinue drug if abnormalities occur
- Therapy should continune for 6–9 months or at least 6 months after sputum cultures are negative
- If compliance is a problem, intermittent dosing with 600 mgl/day, 2–3 day/week can be tried after 1–2 months of initial therapy

PATIENT EDUCATION:
- Drug may cause urine, sweat, tears, feces, saliva to turn red-orange; contact lens may be permanently discolored
- Drug may interfere with oral contraceptives, so women should use alternative contraceptive
- Avoid alcohol
- Need to take drug as directed for 6–9 months

Sargramostim (GM-CSF)

BRAND NAMES:
- Leukine, Prokine

ACTION:
- Recombinant granulocyte-macrophage colony-stimulating factor stimulates growth and differentiation of granulocytes and macrophages, thus preventing febrile neutropenia

INDICATIONS:
- To accelerate myeloid recovery after bone marrow suppressive chemotherapy during bone marrow transplantation in patients with non-Hodgkin's lymphoma, Hodgkin's disease, and acute lymphocytic leukemia; and in patients who have failed engraftment after transplantation.
- Is being tested in clinical trials for AIDS-related non-Hodgkin's lymphoma to hasten granulocyte recovery; also used to prevent neutropenia in patients receiving ganciclovir

CONTRAINDICATIONS:
- Excessive leukemic myeloid blast cells in bone marrow or peripheral blood >10%
- Known hypersensitivity to GM-CSF or yeast

- Patients with HIV disease not receiving antiretroviral therapy, since GM-CSF will hasten replication of HIV-infected monocytes/macrophages
- Use with caution in patients with preexisting peripheral edema, capillary leak syndrome, cardiovascular disease, pleural or pericardial effusions, as drug may worsen fluid retention
- Use with caution in pregnant or breast-feeding women

DOSAGE:
- After autologous bone marrow transplantation: 250 µg/m2/day as 2 hour infusion X 14 days, beginning 2–4 hours after bone marrow infusion
- Engraftment failure: 250 µg/m2/day as 2 hour infusion X 14 days; can repeat if no engraftment, 7 days later; then, if no engraftment, try 500 µg/m2/day X 14 days
- Postchemotherapy (investigational): 250 µg/m^2 sc qd X 10–14 days or 20 µg/kg SC q d X 10 days

ADMINISTRATION:
- Reconstitute aseptically using sterile water for injection. DO NOT SHAKE

- For IV use, further dilute in 0.9% normal saline USP. If final concentration is < 10 µg/mL, add human albumin 0.1% to prevent adsorption to IV tubing. 0.1% albumin is prepared by adding 1 mL human albumin per 1 mL 0.9% sodium chloride (i.e., 5% human albumin in 50 mL 0.9% sodium chloride injection USP). Please refer to package insert

DRUG INTERACTIONS:
- Drugs that potentiate myeloproliferation: lithium, corticosteroids; use together with caution

ADVERSE EFFECTS:
- Fever
- Diarrhea
- Fluid retention, dyspnea
- Edema, capillary leak syndrome
- Supraventricular arrhythmias
- Headache, myalgia, arthralgia
- Pleural, pericardial effusions
- Asthenia, malaise, bone pain
- Local injection site reactions
- Rash

SPECIAL NURSING CONSIDERATIONS:
- Do NOT administer drug within 24 hours preceding or following chemotherapy, or within 12 hours preceding or following radiotherapy

- Monitor patients with preexisting lung disease carefully during and after treatment, especially when drug is given IV (granulocytes are sequested in the pulmonary circulation)
- Monitor body weight and hydration status closely during and after drug infusion
- Fever, asthenia, headache, and bone pain are well controlled with acetaminophen
- Monitor hepatic or renal function studies baseline and 2 X/week in patients with dysfunction
- Monitor CBC, neutrophil count 2 X/week to ensure WBC, neutrophil count does not exceed 50,000/mm^3 (WBC) and 20,000/mm^3 (ANC)

PATIENT EDUCATION:
- Self-administration technique
- Report rash, edema, difficulty breathing immediately

Spectinomycin Dihydrochloride

BRAND NAME:
- Trobicin

ACTION:
- Bacteriostatic antibiotic, inhibits bacterial protein

INDICATIONS:
- Uncomplicated gonorrhea caused by *Neisseria gonorrhoeae,* for patients allergic to, or who do not respond to, penicillins, cephalosporins, or probenecid, or who are allergic to tetracycline or are unlikely to be compliant with a multidose regimen

CONTRAINDICATIONS:
- Prior hypersensitivity

DOSAGE:
- *Adult:* 2 gm X 1 (uncomplicated); 2 gm bid X 3–7 days (disseminated)
- *Children:* 40 mg/kg (max 2 gm) but safety has not been established

ADMINISTRATION:
- Deep IM into upper outer quadrant of gluteal muscle using 20 gauge needle
- Available as 2 gm or 4 gm vials

DRUG INTERACTIONS:
- None

ADVERSE EFFECTS:
- Pain at injection site
- *Occasional:*
  —Urticaria
  —Fever, chills
  —Rash

—Nervousness
—Pruritis
—Insomnia
—Dizziness
—Headache
—Nausea. vomiting
- *Rare:*
—Anaphylaxis

SPECIAL NURSING CONSIDERATIONS:
- Centers for Disease Control (CDC) recommend as first-line therapy a single IM dose of cefriaxone followed by doxycycline
- When spectinomycin is used, it should be followed by oral doxycyline or tetracycline therapy to eliminate coexisting chlamydial and mycoplasmic infections
- All patients should be tested (serologic) for syphilis when drug is given and at 3 months since drug may mask or delay symptoms
- Anaphylaxis rare but be alert; have accessible O_2, corticosteroids, epinephrine; maintain patent airway

PATIENT EDUCATION:
- Report any signs/symptoms of hypersensitivity immediately
- Safe sexual practices to prevent reinfection

Spiramycin

BRAND NAME:
- (Rovamycine) (investigational)

ACTION:
- Macrolide antibiotic, active against parasites

INDICATIONS:
- Toxoplasmosis, chronic cryptosporidiosis

CONTRAINDICATIONS:
- Hypersensitivity to drug

DOSAGE:
- Toxoplasmosis: 2–4 gm q d; children 50–100 mg/kg/day X 3–4 weeks
- Cryptosporidiosis: 2–4 gm q d in 2 divided doses

ADMINISTRATION:
- Oral

DRUG INTERACTIONS:
- Unknown

ADVERSE EFFECTS:
- Nausea, vomiting, epigastric pain, skin sensitization, bronchial asthma (rare)

SPECIAL NURSING CONSIDERATIONS/ PATIENT EDUCATION:
- Similar to erythromycin
- Available from CDC for use on a compassionate IND

Drug Profiles

Stavudine (D$_4$T)

BRAND NAME:
- Investigational agent

ACTION:
- Antiretroviral agent (nucleoside analogue)

INDICATIONS:
- Patients with HIV disease who have failed or are intolerant to zidovudine and didanosine

CONTRAINDICATIONS:
- Use cautiously, if at all, in patients with peripheral neuropathy or hepatic dysfunction

DOSAGE:
- 20–80 mg q d per protocol
- Maximum tolerated dose as well as minimal effective dose as single drug is 2 mg/kg/day

ADMINISTRATION:
- Oral, with or without food

DRUG INTERACTIONS:
- Unknown
- Do not combine with zidovudine, as antagonism may occur

ADVERSE EFFECTS:
- Peripheral neuropathy (high dose)
- Increase liver enzymes
- Myelosuppression

SPECIAL NURSING CONSIDERATIONS:
- For more information on drug, contact Bristol-Myers Squibb (1-800-662-7999)
- Patient responses include 50% or greater increase in CD_4 counts lasting ≥ 1 year in some patients, decrease in p24 antigen levels, weight gain
- Enhances cognitive functioning similar to zidovudine
- Monitor amylase, liver function tests, CBC closely
- Monitor neurological functioning closely

PATIENT EDUCATION:
- Patient should report burning, tingling, numbness in hands or feet immediately
- Per study protocol

Streptomycin Sulfate

BRAND NAME:
- Streptomycin Sulfate

ACTION:
- Aminoglycoside antibacterial agent, inhibits bacterial protein synthesis

INDICATIONS:
- Treatment of *Mycobacterium tuberculosis* in conjunction with at least 1 other drug, second-line agent against *Nocardia, M. Avium* intracellulare, other sensitive organisms

CONTRAINDICATIONS:
- Known hypersensitivity to drug or other aminoglycoside antibiotics
- Pregnant women
- Nursing mothers

DOSAGE:
- *Adult:* 1 gm IM q d X 2–3 months, then 1 gm 2–3 X/week
- *Children:* 20 mg/kg/day in divided doses IM
- Impaired renal function: duration of treatment is modified

ADMINISTRATION:
- Available for injection in 400 mg/mL, 500 mg/ mL, 1 gm, 5 gm vials
- IM deep into large muscle mass, e.g., gluteus in upper outer quadrant of buttock
- Never give IV

DRUG INTERACTIONS:
- Ototoxic drugs (acyclovir, aminoglycosides, amphotericin B, vancomycin): increases risk of ototoxicity, avoid concurrent use if possible
- Succinylcholine, tubercurarine: potentiation of neuromuscular blockade; observe for respiratory depression

ADVERSE EFFECTS:
- Ototoxicity
- Sterile abscesses at injection site
- Nephrotoxicity
- Headache, tremor, lethargy
- Rash, pruritis, fever
- Nausea, vomiting, anorexia
- Transient hepatotoxicity
- Rarely, blood dyscrasias (Increases liver function tests, hepatomegaly)

SPECIAL NURSING CONSIDERATIONS:
- Desired peak serum level 5–25 µg/mL, and trough < 5 µg/mL
- Assess baseline hearing, during therapy, and at completion
- Assess for signs/symptoms of: 8th cranial nerve damage: vestibular (dizziness, nystagmus, vertigo, ataxia), and auditory (tinnitus, roaring in ears, hearing impairment). Change to another agent if signs/symptoms appear
- Assess baseline renal function, and monitor periodically during treatment. Renal dysfunction reversible on drug discontinuation
- Streptomycin discontinued when sputum cultures negative for tuberculosis

PATIENT EDUCATION:
- Report any hearing loss, roaring sounds, ringing in ears or fullness immediately

- Risk of sterile abscesses and need to rotate sites
- Report any signs/symptoms of (super)infection

Sulbactam

BRAND NAME:
- Sulbactam (Investigational)

ACTION:
- Beta-lactamase inhibitor, extends the antimicrobial range of beta-lactam antibiotics

INDICATIONS:
- Often administered with ampicillin or cefoperazone in treating infections involving beta-lactamase production

CONTRAINDICATIONS:
- Hypersensitivity to drug
- Use cautiously in renal dysfunction

DOSAGE:
- Given in a ratio of 1:2 to ampicillin, e.g., sulbactam 0.25–1 gm plus ampicillin 0.5–2 gm IM or IV q 6 hours

ADMINISTRATION:
- IM or IV

DRUG INTERACTIONS:
- Ampicillin: increased antibiotic efficacy
- Cefoperazone: increased efficacy

ADVERSE EFFECTS:
- Pain at injection site (IM)
- Diarrhea
- Phlebitis
- Rash

SPECIAL NURSING CONSIDERATIONS:
- Dose reduce in renal failure
- Investigational

PATIENT EDUCATION:
- Report drug side effects

Sulfadiazine

BRAND NAME:
- Microsulfon

ACTION:
- Antibacterial sulfonamide

INDICATIONS:
- Used with pyrimethamine in the treatment of toxoplasmosis, and with quinine sulfate and pyrimethamine for treatment of uncomplicated malaria resistant to chloroquine
- Used alone in the treatment of nocardiosis, and as prophylaxis of recurrent rheumatic fever

CONTRAINDICATIONS:
- Known hypersensitivity to sulfonamides
- Patients with porphyria
- Pregnant women or breast-feeding mothers
- Use with caution in patients with G6PD deficiency

DOSAGE:
- Toxoplasmosis:
  —*Adults:* 2–8 gm q d in 3–6 divided doses X 6–8 weeks in AIDS patients followed by chronic suppressive therapy at lower doses
  —*Children:* 100–200 mg/kg q d (max 6 gm/day)
- Nocardiosis: adults: 4–8 gm q d X 6 weeks

ADMINISTRATION:
- Orally

DRUG INTERACTIONS:
- Methotrexate: potentiate methotrexate drug effects; use together with caution
- Coumarin anticoagulants: increases anticoagulant effect; monitor closely
- Oral hypoglycemics; increases hypoglycemia; monitor closely
- Phenytoin: increases drug levels; monitor closely

ADVERSE EFFECTS:
- Hypersensitivity reactions: fever 7–10 days after starting drug, rash, pruritis; rarely, Stevens-Johnson syndrome (high fever, severe head-

ache, stomatitis, conjunctivitis, urethritis may precede skin lesions)
- Blood dyscrasias
- Neurotoxicity (psychosis, neuritis)
- Hepatic, renal (crystalluria) dysfunction
- Headache
- Depression, lassitude
- Nausea, vomiting

SPECIAL NURSING CONSIDERATIONS:
- Usual regimen for toxoplasmosis treatment in AIDS patients has > 90% response by 14 days. If no response, brain biopsy of CNS lesion recommended
- Pyrimethamine 100 mg PO bid on day 1 (loading dose), then 50–75 mg PO q d PLUS sulfadiazine 200 mg/kg (4–8 gm) PO q d X 3–6 weeks
- Optimal dose and duration for chronic suppresive therapy unknown. Commonly, pyrimethamine 50 mg PO q d plus sulfadiazine 2 gm PO q d
- Value of folinic acid to lessen pyrimethamine toxicity has not been demonstrated in controlled clinical trials
- Increase fluids to 2–3 L/day to reduce drug precipitation in urinary tract (crystalluria)
- Monitor renal function (BUN, creatinine) baseline and periodically during treatment
- Discontinue drug immediately if rash develops

PATIENT EDUCATION:
- Stop drug and notify physician or nurse if rash develops
- Report all drug side effects
- Importance of long-term therapy

Terconazole

BRAND NAME:
- Terazol 3 vaginal cream 0.8%
- Terazol 7 vaginal cream 0.4%
- Terazol 3 vaginal suppositories 80 mg

ACTION:
- Antifungal agent

INDICATIONS:
- Vulvovaginal candidiasis (moniliasis)

CONTRAINDICATIONS:
- Known hypersensitivity
- Pregnant women in first trimester
- Nursing mothers
- Children

DOSAGE:
- 1 full applicator (5 g) Terazol 3 X 3 days
- 1 full applicator (5 g) Terazol 7 X 7 days
- 1 suppository Terazol 3 X 3 days

ADMINISTRATION:
- Insert full applicator of cream or suppository intravaginally at bedtime

DRUG INTERACTIONS:
- None known

ADVERSE EFFECTS:
- Headache
- Dysmenorrhea
- Abdominal pain
- Pruritis

SPECIAL NURSING CONSIDERATIONS:
- Discontinue drug and do not resume if irritation, fever, chills, or flu-like symptoms develop
- Therapeutic effect not cream or suppositories not affected by menstruation
- If symptoms persist after treatment, culture vaginal flora or test with KOH prep

PATIENT EDUCATION:
- Stop drug and notify nurse or physician if fever, chills, or flu-like symptoms develop
- Remove rubber latex products such as vaginal contraceptive diaphragms prior to treatment

Thiabendazole

BRAND NAME:
- Mintezol

ACTION:
- Antihelminthic agent

INDICATIONS:
- Strongyloidiasis (threadworm)
- Cutaneous larva migrans (creeping eruption)
- Visceral larva migrans
- Trichinosis (invasive stages)

CONTRAINDICATIONS:
- Known hypersensitivity
- Use cautiously in persons with hepatic or renal dysfunction, anemia, malnutrition
- Use in pregnant women or nursing mothers unless benefits outweigh risks

DOSAGE:
- Strongyloides: Adult: 22 mg/kg (max 1.5 gm) PO q 12 hours X 2 days

ADMINISTRATION:
- Available as oral chewable tablet (chewed thoroughly before swallowing)
- Available as suspension
- Administer after meals

DRUG INTERACTIONS:
- Theophylline: may increase thiabendazole levels; monitor for toxicity and dose reduce if needed

ADVERSE EFFECTS:
- Occur 3–4 hours after drug administration, and last 2–8 hours
- Anorexia, nausea, vomiting, dizziness
- Diarrhea, epigastric distress, weariness, drowsiness
- Psychic disturbances
- Giddiness, paresthesia, vertigo
- Hypersensitivity reactions (pruritis, fever, chills, facial flushing, rash, conjunctival injection, angioedema)

SPECIAL NURSING CONSIDERATIONS:
- If hypersensitivity reaction occurs, discontinue drug immediately; DO NOT resume, as erythema multiforme may occur
- CNS side effects are frequent, so patient should avoid driving car, operating heavy machinery since mental alertness may be clouded
- Retreatment often required

PATIENT EDUCATION:
- Avoid activities requiring mental alertness
- Retreatment may be necessary
- Report any change in condition
- Report fever, chills, rash, pruritis immediately

Tioconazole 6.5%

BRAND NAME:
- Vagistat-1

ACTION:
- Broad-spectrum antifungal agent

INDICATIONS:
- Vulvovaginal candidiasis (moniliasis)

CONTRAINDICATIONS:
- Hypersensitivity to imidazole antifungal agents
- Pregnant women unless benefit outweighs risk
- Nursing mothers

DOSAGE:
- 1 prefilled applicator

ADMINISTRATION:
- Use applicator to iinsert medication intravaginally

DRUG INTERACTIONS:
- None known

ADVERSE EFFECTS:
- Burning, itching (6%)
- *Less common:*
  —Irritation, discharge
  —Vulvar edema/swelling

Memory Bank for HIV Medications

—Vaginal pain
—Dysuria
—Burning sensation

SPECIAL NURSING CONSIDERATIONS:
* Negligible systemic absorption
* Safety and effectiveness in diabetics, pregnancy, or children have not been established

PATIENT EDUCATION:
* Take dose at bedtime
* Ointment may interact with rubber or latex products (e.g., condom, vaginal diaphragm) so avoid use/contact for 72 hours

Trazodone Hydrochloride

BRAND NAME:
* Desyrek

ACTION:
* Antidepressant

INDICATIONS:
* Depression

CONTRAINDICATIONS:
* Known hypersensitivity to drug
* Initial phases of myocardial infarction

DOSAGE:
- 150 mg/day in divided doses
- Dose may be increased by 50 mg/day every 3–4 days
- Max dose (outpatients) is 400 mg/day in 4 divided doses
- Max dose (inpatient)is 600 mg/day in divided doses

ADMINISTRATION:
- Take with food or just after a meal
- Dose may be taken at bedtime if drowsy

DRUG INTERACTIONS:
- Digoxin: increased serum digoxin level; assess for toxicity and modify dose prn
- Phenytoin: increased serum phenytoin level; assess for toxicity
- Alcohol: increased CNS depression; avoid concurrent use
- Barbiturates: increased CNS depression; avoid concurrent use

ADVERSE EFFECTS:
- Priapism
- Arrhythmias
- Dry mouth, constipation, blurred vision
- Hypotension
- Drowsiness, dizziness/lightheadedness, fatigue, nervousness
- Muscle aches and pains
- Incoordination

SPECIAL NURSING CONSIDERATIONS:
- Suicide in depressed patients is a worry, and thus only a limited number of tablets should be given at a time
- Optimal antidepressant effects occur in 2 weeks

PATIENT EDUCATION:
- Male patients with prolonged or inappropriate erections should stop the drug and notify their doctor or nurse
- To avoid operating heavy machinery or driving a car if mental or physical ability impaired
- To avoid alcohol, barbiturates, CNS depressants

Trimethoprim Sulfate

BRAND NAMES:
- Trimpex, Proloprirn

ACTION:
- Antibacterial agent. inhibits bacterial synthesis of folic acid

INDICATIONS:
- Urinary tract infections (UTI) caused by *E. Coil, Proteus mirabilis, Klebsiella, Enterobacter*
- Used in treatment of initial episodes of *Pneumocystis carinii* pneumonia (PCP) with dapsone

CONTRAINDICATIONS:
- Megaloblastic anemia due to folate deficiency
- Known hypersensitivity
- Pregnancy
- Nursing mothers
- Use with caution: impaired renal or hepatic function, folate deficiency

DOSAGE:
- UTI: *Adult:* 100 mg PO q 12 hours X 10 days
- PCP: Trimethoprim 20 mg/kg q d in 4 divided doses plus dapsone 100 mg PO q d X 21 days
- Modify dose if renal impairment

ADMINISTRATION:
- Available in 100 mg and 200 mg tablets
- Oral

DRUG INTERACTIONS:
- Phenytoin: increases serum levels; decrease phenytoin dosage

ADVERSE EFFECTS:
- *Common:*
  —Rash, pruritis, appearing 7–14 days after beginning therapy
- *Uncommon:*
  —Bone marrow suppression (rare)
  —Epigastric discomfort
  —Nausea
  —Vomiting
  —Glossitis

SPECIAL NURSING CONSIDERATIONS:
- Less toxic than trimethoprim-sulfamethoxazole
- Monitor CBC baseline
- Use in treatment of PCP is off-label. Use not approved by U.S. Food and Drug Administration
- When used with dapsone for initial epidoses of PCP, most patients show improvement within 6 days

PATIENT EDUCATION:
- Report drug side effects
- Report increase in fatigue, pallor, other signs of anemia
- Need to comply with treatment regime for PCP

Trimethoprim and Sulfamethoxazole (TMP-SMX) Co-Trimoxazole

BRAND NAMES:
- Bacrim, Bactrim DS, Cotrim, Septra, Septra DS, Sulfamethoprim, Sulfamethoprim DS

ACTION:
- Sulfonamide antibiotic; prevents bacterial and protozoal replication by inhibiting folic acid synthesis

INDICATIONS:
- *Pneumocystis carinii* pneumonia (PCP)

- Urinary tract infection (caused by *E. coli,* Klebsiella, Enterobacter)
- *Shigella* enteritis

CONTRAINDICATIONS:
- Known hypersensitivity to trimethoprim or sulfonamides
- Folate deficiency anemia, renal failure, or porphyria
- Pregnant or breast-feeding women
- Use with caution in G6PD deficiency, and use reduced drug dose

DOSAGE:
- PCP:
  Adult:
  —Prophylaxis: TMP-SMX 1 double strength (DS) tablet (TMP 160 SMX 800 mg) PO q d or 3 X/week
  —Treatment: TMP-SMX 2 DS tablets PO 4 X/day (total 15–20 mg/kg TMP/day oral or IV) X 21 days
  Children:
  —20 mg/kg TMP/day PO, in 4 equally divided doses; IV dose is 15–20 mg/kg/day in 3–4 divided doses
- UTI, Shigellosis:
  Adult: 1 TMP-SMX DS tab or 2 tabs TMP-SMX q 12 hours X 10–14 days (UTI) or 5 days (Shigellosis)

Children: 8 mg/kg TMP and 40 mg/kg SMX per
24 hours in 2 divided doses q 12 hours x 10
days (UTI) or 5 days (shigellosis)
- MODIFY DOSE IN RENAL IMPAIRMENT

ADMINISTRATION:
- Oral: take with 8 oz. of water
- IV: administer over 1–1.5 hours

DRUG INTERACTIONS:
- Warfarin: increased prothrombin time (PT);
  monitor PT closely, and decrease warfarin dose
  as needed
- Sulfonureas: increased hypoglycemic effect;
  monitor blood glucose closely, and reduce
  sulfonurea dose as needed
- Phenytoin: increased and prolonged serum
  phenytoin serum levels; monitor level closely
  and reduce dose as needed
- Methotrexate: increased methotrexate level and
  potential toxicity (bone marrow depression,
  mucositis); monitor levels, or decrease
  methotrexate dose

ADVERSE EFFECTS:
- Increased adverse effects seen in HIV-infected
  patients:
  —Rash, skin reactions
  —Fever
  —Leukopenia
  —Increased liver function tests (amino-
  transaminase)

SPECIAL NURSING CONSIDERATIONS:

- Co-trimazole has 1 mg TMP for every 5 mg SMX
- Most cost-effective therapy for PCP, but increased risk of toxicity and intolerance in HIVinfected patients; cure rate > 40–50% for initial episodes PCP
- Initial treatment should be followed by prophylaxis therapy (secondary prevention)
- Prophylaxis should be given to patients with CD counts < 200/mm^3
- Skin reactions ranging from mild maculopapular rash with urticaria, pruritis, to erythema multiforme, exfoliative dermatitis and Stevens-Johnson syndrome: usually occurs 7–14 days after beginning drug therapy
- Monitor CBC baseline, and periodically during therapy
- Monitor serum BUN, creatinine, baseline and during therapy

PATIENT EDUCATION:

- Discontinue drug and notify doctor or nurse if rash develops
- Assess for and report infection, bleeding, increased fatigue, and any change(s) in condition
- Take drug with at least 8 oz. of water; increased total oral intake to 2–3 L/24 hours

Trimetrexate Gluconate

BRAND NAME:
- Investigational agent

ACTION:
- Antimetabolite agent, inhibits difolate reductase preventing cell replication; inhibits growth of some parasites (i.e., *Pneumoncystis carinii* pneumonia, toxoplasmosis)

INDICATIONS:
- Available under a treatment IND for treatment of patients with *Pneumocystis carinii* pneumonia in the hospital who have intolerance to both cotrimoxazole and pentamidine

CONTRAINDICATIONS:
- Myelosuppression
- Pregnant women

DOSAGE:
- Per protocol
- May need to dose reduce if hepatic dysfunction

ADMINISTRATION:
- IV
- Must be given with leukovorin (folinic acid) rescue

DRUG INTERACTIONS:
- Myelosuppressive drugs (zidovudine): AVOID concurrent use
- Nephrotoxic drugs: potentially increase renal damage: AVOID concurrent use

ADVERSE EFFECTS:
- Myelosuppression (MAY BE LIFE THREATENING), especially leukopenia, thrombocytopenia
- Nausea, vomiting
- Stomatitis
- Diarrhea
- Increased SGOT

SPECIAL NURSING CONSIDERATIONS:
- Intolerance to co-trimoxazole:
  —Platelet count < 50,000/mm^3, ANC < 500/mm^3 X 2
  —Mucocutaneous blistering rash
  —Hepatitis
- Intolerance to pentamidine:
  —Platelet count < 50,000/mm^3, ANC ≤ 500/ mm^3 X 2
  —Nephrotoxicity with serum creatinine > 3 mg/dL
  —Hypotension: SBP < 90 requiring fluids
  —Dysglycemia: BS < 40 mg/dL or hyperglycemia requiring treatment
  —Pancreatitis
- Monitor LFTs baseline and throughout treatment

—Contact manufacturer (Michigan), Warner Lambert (1-800-426-7527) or National Information Center for Orphan Drugs and Rare Diseases (1-800-336-4797)

PATIENT EDUCATION:
- Self-assess for side effects
- Self-administration of antiemetics

VANCOMYCIN HYDROCHLORIDE

BRAND NAMES:
- Vancocin, Lyphocin, Vancor

ACTION:
- Antibacterial aagent, prevents bacterial wall synthesis

INDICATIONS:
- Severe staphylococcal infections, including those unresponsive to penicillin, cephalosporins
- Pseudomembranous colitis

CONTRAINDICATIONS:
- Known hypersensitivity
- Previous hearing loss

- Use with caution if renal dysfunction, and modify dose
- Pregnancy unless benefit outweighs risk

DOSAGE
Adult:
- IV: 500 mg–1 gm q 12 hours
- Oral: via nasogastric (NG) tube for pseudomembranous colitis: capsules or powder 0.5–2 gm q d in 3–4 divided doses X 7–10 days

ADMINISTRATION:
- PO, IV over 1 hour
- NEVER IM as causes tissue necrosis

DRUG INTERACTIONS:
- Amikacin, gentamicin, kanamycin, tobramycin, amphotericin B, cisplatin: increase nephrotoxicity; don't use together if possible

ADVERSE EFFECTS:
- Ototoxicity
- Nephrotoxicity Phlebitis
- Superinfection
- Hypersensitivity reactions (5–10%): nausea, chills, fever, urticaria, rash

SPECIAL NURSING CONSIDERATIONS:
- Monitor serum BUN and creatine baseline and throughout therapy
- Most patients show response in 48–72 hours of beginning IV therapy

* Report rash
* Report decrease in hearing, tinnitus, vertigo, dizziness

Vinblastine Sulfate

BRAND NAMES:
* Velban, Velsar

ACTION:
* Antineoplastic agent; inhibits mitosis, thus preventing cell replication

INDICATIONS:
* Kaposi's sarcoma (KS)
* Lymphoma
* Testicular cancer

CONTRAINDICATIONS:
* Known hypersensitivity Concurrent infection
* Leukopenia, thrombocytopenia

DOSAGE:
* IV: 0.05–0.1 mg/kg or 3 mg/m^2 q 1–2 weeks
* Intralesional: 0.01–0.1 mg/lesion
* Modify dose if obstructive jaundice or hepatic dysfunction

ADMINISTRATION:
- IV: vesicant must be given slow IVP via freely flowing, patent IV with excellent blood return confirmed throughout—USE EXPERT TECHNIQUE in administration to avoid EXTRAVASATION
  —If drug infiltrates
    –Aspirate any remaining drug from IV tubing
    –Administer hyaluronidase into area of infiltration
    –Apply heat
    –Refer to institutional guidelines for management of vesicant extravasation
- Intralesional: 0.01 mg in 0.1 mL sterile water
- Use chemotherapy handling precautions (see Appendix I)
- DRUG SHOULD BE ADMINISTERED ONLY BY A NURSE SKILLED IN CHEMOTHERAPY ADMINISTRATION and should be administered according to institutional guidelines for chemotherapy administration

DRUG INTERACTIONS:
- Phenytoin: decreased anticonvulsant activity
- Methotrexate: vinblastine increases cell uptake of methotrexate when given prior to methotrexate

ADVERSE EFFECTS:
- Skin necrosis if drug extravasates (infiltrates)
- Bone marrow depression 4–10 days after drug given (neutropenia, thrombocytopenia), especially if larger doses given
- Alopecia, peripheral neuropathy with long-term use
- Rare stomatitis, nausea, vomiting

SPECIAL NURSING CONSIDERATIONS:
- Dose-limiting toxicity: myelosuppression
- Regimens used in KS:
  —Vinblastine 0.05–0.1 mg/kg or 3 mg/m^2 weekly IV (absolute neutrophil count > 1000/mm^3): 25–30% response
  —Vincristine 2 mg/week IV alternating with vinblastine 0.1 mg/kg or 3 mg/m^2 every other week; 45% response

SPECIAL NURSING CONSIDERATIONS:
- Prior to drug administration:
  —Review institutional policy and procedure on administration of vesicant chemotherapy
  —Assess WBC > 4000/mm^3 unless receiving granluocyte-colony-stimulating factor
  —Assess signs/symptoms peripheral neuropathy, deep tendon reflexes
  —Assess tolerance of prior chemotherapy (if applicable)
  —Assess patency of IV (if in doubt, RESTART IV)

—Consider implanted subcutaneous venous access port if patient has poor venous access
—USE SAFE HANDLING PRACTICES (see Appendix I)

PATIENT EDUCATION:
- Report any stinging, burning during IV drug adminstration immediately
- Alopecia is temporary, and hair will regrow
- Assess signs/symptoms of infection and report immediately
- Report signs/symptoms of neuropathy: paresthesias, burning in hands or feet, sensory loss, difficulty walking

Vincristine Sulfate

BRAND NAME:
- Oncovin

ACTION:
- Antineoplastic agent, inhibits mitosis, thus preventing malignant cell replication

INDICATIONS:
- Acute leukemia
- Used in treatment of Kaposi's sarcoma (KS), lymphoma, other malignancies

CONTRAINDICATIONS:

- Known hypersensitivity
- Charcot-Marie-Tooth syndrome (syndrome of progressive muscle atrophy of neuropathic origin)

DOSAGE:

- 1.4–2 mg IVP q 1–4 weeks
- Modify dose in hepatic failure

ADMINISTRATION:

- IVP through patent, freely flowing IV with blood return confirmed throughout
- DRUG IS A VESICANT—extravasation may cause severe tissue necrosis—USE EXPERT TECHNIQUE in administration to AVOID EXTRAVASATION
- NEVER ADMINISTER INTRATHECALLY
- Use chemotherapy handling precautions (see Appendix I)
- DRUG SHOULD BE ADMINISTERED ONLY BY NURSES SKILLED IN CHEMOTHERAPY ADMINISTRATION, and should be administered according to institutional guidelines for chemotherapy administration

DRUG INTERACTIONS:

- Neurotoxic drugs; additive neurotoxicity; use cautiously
- Digoxin; decrease digoxin serum level possible; monitor closely

- Methotrexate: vincristine increases cell uptake of methotrexate when given prior to methotrexate

ADVERSE EFFECTS:
- Skin necrosis if drug extravasates (infiltrates)
- Peripheral neuropathy (paresthesia)
- Cranial neuropathy (constipation, diplopia) Alopecia

SPECIAL NURSING CONSIDERATIONS:
- Drug not myelosuppressive
- Regimens used in KS:
  —Vincristine 1.5–2 mg/week IV: 20–60% response
  —Vincristine 2 mg/week IV alternating vinblastine 0.1 mg/kg or 3 mg/m^2 every other week IV; 45% response
  —Vincristine 2 mg IV and bleomycin 10 u/m^2 IV q 14 days; ~ 100% response pulmonary KS
  —ABV:

  doxorubicin 10–20 mg/m^2 IV ⎫ q 14 days;
  bleomycin 10 u/m^2 IV   ⎬ response may be
  vincristine 1.0–2.0 mg IV   ⎭ as high as 87%

- Prior to drug administration:
  —Review institutional policy and procedure on administration of vesicant chemotherapy
  —Assess WBC > 4000/mm^3 unless receiving granulocyte-colony-stimulating factor

Memory Bank for HIV Medications

—Assess signs/symptoms peripheral neuropathy, deep tendon reflexes
—Assess tolerance of prior chemotherapy (if applicable)
—Assess patency of IV (if in doubt, RESTART IV)
—Consider implanted subcutaneous venous access port if patient has poor venous access
—USE SAFE HANDLING PRACTICES (see Appendix I)

PATIENT EDUCATI ON:
- Report any stinging or burning during drug administration immediately
- Self-assess and report numbness, weakness, myalgias, difficulty walking or buttoning shirt, double vision, constipation
- Measures to prevent constipation

Zalcitabine (Dideoxycytidine, ddC)

BRAND NAME:
- HIVID

ACTION:
- Antiretroviral agent; nucleoside analogue that inhibits the enzyme reverse transcriptase, thus preventing viral replication

INDICATIONS:
- In combination with zidevudine, for the treatment of adult patients with advanced HIV infection (CD < 300 cells/mm^3) or who show clinical or immunologoc deterioration on zidovudine alone

CONTRAINDICATIONS:
- Known hypersensitivity to the drug
- Use with extreme caution, if at all, in patients with preexisting peripheral neuropathy
- Use with extreme caution, if at all, in patients with history of pancreatitis, or known risk factors
- Use with extreme caution in patients with CD$_4$ counts < 50 cells/rnm^3 as high risk of developing penpheral neuropathy
- Breast-feeding mothers

DOSAGE:
- 0.750 mg q 8 hours together with zidovudine 200 mg q 8 hours
- Renal insufficiency: dose-reduce based on creatinine clearance: 10–40 mg/mL– 0.750 mg q 12 hours; < 10 mg/mL = 0.750 mg q 24 hours
- Hepatic dysfunction: monitor closely, may require dose modification or drug discontinuance

ADMINISTRATION:
- Orally

DRUG INTERACTIONS:
- IV pentamidine: fatal pancreatitis has occurred; HOLD ZALCITABINE during IV pentamidine therapy
- Drugs causing peripheral neuropathy (e.g., chloramphenicol, cisplatin, dapsone, hydralazine, isoniazid, metronidazole, phenytoin, ribavarin, vincrlstine): AVOID concomitant use
- Didanosine: AVOID concurrent use
- Drugs causing renal insufficiency (e.g., amphotericin, loscarnet, aminoglycosides): monitor renal function, and dose may need to be reduced

ADVERSE EFFECTS:
- Peripheral neuropathy (17–31% of patients)*
- Pancreatitis (<1% of patients)*
- Oral ulcers*
- Increased liver function tests (LFTs)*
- Nausea, dysphagia, anorexia
- Rash, pruritis
- Headache, fever
- Arthralglas, myalgias
- Fatigue
- Rare: esophageal ulcers, cardiomyopathy/ CHF, anaphylaxis*

*Require dose modification or drug discontinuance

SPECIAL NURSING CONSIDERATIONS:
- Baseline CBC, chemistries should be done prior to beginning therapy, and periodically during treatment
- Baseline triglycerides and serum amylase should be determined for patients with prior history of pancreatitis, increased amylase, on total peripheral nutrition (TPN), or with a history of alcohol abuse
- Severe peripheral neuropathy can be disabling, and risk is greater in patients with advanced disease. Drug continuance should be evaluated if signs/symptoms develop
- Discontinue both zalcitabine and zidovudine if patient develops increased LFTs, or other serious adverse effects; physician may reintroduce drugs at lower doses once symptoms resolved

PATIENT EDUCATION:
- Drugs not a cure for HIV but prevent viral replication
- Long-term effects of this combined therapy are unknown
- Report all changes in condition (physical and mental)
- Signs/symptoms of neuropathy (numbness and burning dysesthesia of distal extremities, and, if continue on drug, sharp shooting pains or severe continuous burning): patient should report these immediately

- Signs/symptoms of pancreatitis (nausea, vomiting, abdominal pain): stop drug and see provider immediately

Zidovudine (AZT)

BRAND NAME:
- Retrovir

ACTION:
- Antiretroviral agent; nucleoside analogue that inhibits the enzyme reverse transcriptase, thus preventing viral replication

INDICATIONS:
- Management of HIV infection in patients with CD_4 counts < $200/mm^3$, with or without symptoms. May be combined in alternating fashion with other antiretroviral agents to lessen toxicity; use in patients with CD_4 counts $200–500/mm^3$ is controversial (Consensus Statement, 1993)

CONTRAINDICATIONS:
- Known hypersensitivity to the drug
- Breast-feeding mothers
- Use when risk outweighs benefit in pregnant women

DOSAGE:
- *Adults:* 100 mg PO 5 X/day or 200 mg tid (asymptomatic) to 6 X/day (symptomatic); 1–2 mg/kg IV q 4 hours X ,5–6 (if unable to take PO)
- *Children:* 180 mg/m^2 q 6 hours (max 200 mg q 6 hours)

ADMINISTRATION:
- Oral; available as 100 mg capsules or syrup (10 mg/mL); IV as needed when unable to use oral route

DRUG INTERACTIONS:
- Acyclovir: increased neurotoxicity (profound drowsiness, lethargy); monitor closely
- Alfa interferon: synergism, and increased AZT effect: monitor toxicity closely
- Amphotericin, dapsone: increased bone marrow toxicity: monitor CBC closely
- Co-trimoxazole: possible increased anemia, neutropenia risk; may need to hold AZT during high-dose co-trimoxazole therapy
- Ganciclovir: increased hematologic toxicity; avoid concurrent use
- Methadone: increased AZT metabolism: monitor toxicity closely when beginning methadone or increasing dose
- Nephrotoxic, cytotoxic, or myelosuppressive drugs: potential I in zidovudine toxicity; use with caution and monitor closely

- Nephrotoxic, cytotoxic, or myelosuppressive drugs: potential I in zidovudine toxicity; use with caution and monitor closely
- Probenecid: increased serum concentrations of zidovudine; use with caution and assess for increased zidovudine toxicity; dose-reduce zidovudine as needed
- Ribavarin: antagonism; do not use together
- Sulfadiazine/pyrimethamine: decreased AZT clearance with increased bone marrow toxicity; monitor CBC closely

ADVERSE EFFECTS:
- Anemia (macrocytic, megaloblastic), usually occurring 4–6 weeks after initiation of therapy
- Granulocytopenia
- Nausea
- Headache
- *Less common:*
  —Asthenia, malaise. somnolence, restlessness
  —GI/abdominal pain, diarrhea, anorexia, myalgia
  —Rash, pigmentation of nails

SPECIAL NURSING CONSIDERATIONS:
- Toxicity worse in patients with CD_4 counts $< 200/mm^3$
- Monitor hemaglobin/hematocrit, and transfuse as ordered. Some patients may respond to erythropoietin (epoetin). Drug may be held for

- Assess WBC, absolute neutrophil count (ANC), signs/symptoms of infection. Drug will need to be held if ANC < 750/mm^3, or reduction of > 50% from baseline. Patient may require addition of hematopoietic growth factor (G-CSF, GM-CSF) or change to another antiretroviral agent
- Assess for increased drug toxicity in patients with impaired renal or hepatic function
- Assess signs/symptoms of myalgia. muscle weakness in patients receiving long-term zidovudine

PATIENT EDUCATION:
- Take drug exactly as prescribed
- Drug does not kill HIV virus, but prevents replication
- Report signs/symptoms of myalgia, muscle weakness
- Assess signs/symptoms of infection, and report immediately

APPENDIX I

Recommendations for Handling Cytotoxic Agents: National Study Commission on Cytotoxic Exposure, Occupational Safety and Health Administration (OSHA), September 1987

PREAMBLE

The mutagenic, carcinogenic, and local irritant properties of many cytotoxic agents are well established and pose a hazard to the health of occupationally exposed individuals. These potential hazards necessitate special attention to the procedures utilized in the handling, preparation and administration of these drugs, and the proper disposal of residues and wastes. These recommendations are intended to provide information for the protection of personnel participating in the clinical process of chemotherapy. It is the responsibility of institutional and private health care providers to adopt and use appropriate procedures for protection and safety.

I. Environmental Protection

1. Preparation of cytotoxic agents should be performed in a Class 11 biological safety cabinet located in an area with minimal traffic

and air turbulence. Class 11 Type A cabinets
are the minimal requirement. Class 11 cabinets
that are exhausted to the outside are preferred.
2. The biological safety cabinet must be certified
by qualified personnel at least annually or any
time the cabinet is physically moved.

II. Operator Protection
1. Disposable surgical latex gloves are recommended for all procedures involving cytotoxic
agents.
2. Gloves should routinely be changed approximately every 30 minutes when working steadily
with cytotoxic agents. Gloves should be
removed immediately after overt contamination.
3. Protective barrier garments should be worn for
all procedures involving the preparation and
disposal of cytotoxic agents. These garments
should have a closed front, long sleeves, and a
closed cuff (either elastic or knit).
4. Protective garments must not be worn outside
the work area.

III. Techniques and Precautions for Use in the
Class II Biological Safety Cabinet
1. Special techniques and precautions must be
utilized because of the vertical (downward)
laminar airflow.
2. Clean surfaces of the cabinet using 70%
alcohol and a disposable towel before and after
preparation. Discard towel into a hazardous
chemical waste container.

3. Prepare the work surface of the biological safety cabinet by covering it with a plastic-backed absorbent pad. This pad should be changed when the cabinet is cleaned or after a spill.
4. The biological safety cabinet should be operated with the blower on, 24 hours per day—7 days a week. Where the biological safety cabinet is utilized infrequently (e.g., 1 or 2 times weekly) it may be turned off after thoroughly cleaning all interior surfaces. Turn on the blower 15 minutes before beginning work in the cabinet.
5. Drug preparations must be performed only with the view screen at the recommended access opening. Professionally accepted practices concerning the aseptic preparation of injectable products should be followed.
6. All materials needed to complete the procedure should be placed into the biological safety cabinet before beginning work to avoid interruptions of cabinet airflow. Allow a 2 or 3 minute period before beginning work for the unit to purge itself of airborne contaminants.
7. The proper procedures for use in the biological safety cabinet differ from those used in the horizontal laminar hood because of the nature of the airflow pattern. Clean air descends through the work zone from the top of the

cabinet toward the work surface. As it descends, the air is split, with some leaving through the rear perforation and some leaving through the front perforation.

8. The least efficient area of the cabinet in terms of product and personnel protection is within 3 inches of the sides near the front opening, and work should not be performed in these areas.

9. Entry into and exit from the cabinet should be in a direct manner perpendicular to the face of the cabinet. Rapid movements of the hands in the cabinet and laterally through the protective air barrier should be avoided.

IV. Compounding Procedures and Techniques

1. Hands must be washed thoroughly before gloving and after gloves are removed,

2. Care must be taken to avoid puncturing of gloves and possible self-inoculation.

3. Syringes and IV sets with Luer-lock fittings should be used whenever possible to avoid spills due to disconnection.

4. To minimize aerosolization, vials containing cytotoxic agents should be vented with a hydrophobic filter to equalize internal pressure, or utilize negative pressure technique.

5. Before opening ampules, care should be taken to ensure that no liquid remains in the tip of the ampule. A sterile disposable sponge should be wrapped around the neck of the ampule to

reduce aerosolization. Ampules should be broken in a direction away from the body.

6. For sealed vials, final drug measurement should be performed prior to removing the needle from the stopper of the vial and after the pressure has been equalized.

7. A closed collection vessel should be available in the biological safety cabinet or the original vial may be used to hold discarded excess drug solutions.

8. Cytotoxic agents should be properly labeled to identify the need for caution in handling (e.g., "Chemotherapy: Dispose of Properly").

9. The final prepared dosage form should be protected from leakage or breakage by being sealed in a transparent plastic container labeled "Do Not Open, If Contents Appear To Be Broken."

V. Precautions for Administration
1. Disposable surgical latex gloves should be worn during administration of cytotoxic agents. Hands must be washed thoroughly before gloving and after gloves are removed.

2. Protective **barrier garments may be worn.** Such garments should **have a closed front,**

long sleeves, and a closed cuff (either elastic or knit).

3. Syringes and IV sets with Luer-lock fittings should be used whenever possible.

4. Special care must be taken in priming IV sets. The distal tip or needle cover must be removed before priming. Priming can be performed into a sterile, alcohol-dampened gauze sponge. Other acceptable methods of priming such as closed receptacles (e.g., evacuated containers) or backfilling of IV sets may be utilized. Do not prime sets or syringes into the sink or any open receptacle.

VI. Disposal Procedures
1. Place contaminated materials in a leakproof, puncture-proof container appropriately marked as hazardous chemical waste. These containers should be suitable to collect bottles, vials, gloves, disposable gowns, and other materials used in the preparation and administration of cytotoxic agents.

2. Contaminated needles, syringes, sets, and tubing should be disposed of intact. In order to prevent aerosolization, needles and syringes should not be clipped.

3. Cytotoxic drug waste should be transported according to the institutional procedures for hazardous material.
4. There is insufficient information to recommend any preferred method for disposal of cytotoxic drug waste.
  4.1   One acceptable method for disposal of hazardous waste is by incineration in an Environmental Protection Agency (EPA) permitted hazardous waste incinerator.
  4.2   Another acceptable method of disposal is by burial at an EPA permitted hazardous waste site.
  4.3   A licensed hazardous waste disposal company may be consulted for information concerning available methods of disposal in the local area.

VII.   Personnel Policy Recommendations

1. Personnel involved in any aspect of the handling of cytotoxic agents must receive an orientation to the agents, including their known risks, and special training in safe handling procedures.
2. Access to the compounding area must be limited to authorized personnel.
3. Personnel working with these agents should be supervised regularly to insure compliance with procedures.
4. Acute exposures must be documented, and the employee referred for medical examination.

5. Personnel should refrain from applying cosmetics in the work area. Cosmetics may provide a source of prolonged exposure if contaminated.
6. Eating, drinking, chewing gum, smoking, or storing food in areas where cytotoxic agents are handled should be prohibited. Each of these can be a source of ingestion if they are accidentally contaminated.

VIII. Monitoring Procedures
1. Policies and procedures to monitor the equipment and operating techniques of personnel handling cytotoxic agents should be implemented and performed on a regular basis with appropriate documentation. Specific methods of monitoring should be developed to meet the complexities of the function.
2. It is recommended that personnel involved in the preparation of cytotoxic agents be given periodic health examinations in accordance with institutional policy.

IX. Procedures for Acute Exposure or Spills

1. ACUTE EXPOSURE
    1.1   Overtly contaminated gloves or outer garments should be removed immediately.
    1.2   Hands must be washed after removing gloves. Some cytotoxic agents have been documented to penetrate gloves.

1.3   In case of skin contact with a cytotoxic drug product, the affected area should be washed thoroughly with soap and water. Refer for medical attention as soon as possible.
1.4   For eye exposure, flush **affected eye** with copious amounts of **water, and refer for medical** attention immediately.

2. SPILLS
2.1   All personnel involved in the clean-up of a spill should wear protective barrier garments (e.g., gloves, gowns.). These garments and other materials used in the process should be disposed of properly.
2.2   Double gloving is recommended for cleaning up spills.

POSITION STATEMENT: The Handling of Cytotoxic Agents by Women Who Are Pregnant, Attempting to Conceive, or Breast Feeding

There are substantial data regarding the mutagenic, teratogenic, and abortifacient properties of certain cytotoxic agents, both in animals and in humans who have received therapeutic doses of these agents. Additionally, the scientific literature suggests a possible association of occupational exposure to certain cytotoxic agents during the first trimester of pregnancy with fetal loss or malformation. These data suggest the need for caution when women who are pregnant, or attempting to conceive, handle cytotoxic agents. Incidentally, there is no evidence relating male exposure to cytotoxic agents with adverse fetal outcome, There are no studies that address the possible risk associated with the occupational exposure to cytotoxic agents and the passage of these agents into breast milk. Nevertheless, it is prudent that women who are breast feeding should exercise caution in handing cytotoxic agents. Compliance with all procedures for safe handling, such as those recommended by the Commission, will minimize the potential for exposure. Personnel should be provided with information to make an individual decision. This information should be provided in written form, and it is advisable that a statement of understanding be signed. It is essential to refer to individual state right-to know laws to ensure compliance.

—Approved by the National Study Commission on Cytotoxic Exposure, September 1987.

APPENDIX II

Resources for Indigent Patients

DRUG	RESOURCE	DESCRIPTION
acyclovir (Zovirax)	Burroughs Wellcome 1-800-722-9294	Financial assistance program
didanosine (Videx, ddI)	Bristol-Myers 1-800-788-0123	Reimbursement help line Temporary assistance
epoetin (Procrit)	Ortho Biotech Inc. 1-800-553-358	Financial assistance; cost sharing; reimbursement
filgrastim (Neupogen, G-CSF)	Amgen 1-800-272-9376	Reimbursement hotline safety net program
fluconazole (Diflucan)	Pfizer 1-800-869-9979	Financial assistance
Foscarnet (Foscar)	Astra Pharmaceuticals 1-800-488-3247	Assurance program; Financial assistance, reimbursement information

ganciclovir (Cytovene)	Syntex 1-800-444-4200	Provisional assistance program
interferon-alfa (Roferon-A)	Roche Laboratories 1-800-227-7448	Cost assistance program; Reimbursement information
octreotide (Sandostatin)	Sandoz Pharmaceuticals 1-800-772-7556	Reimbursement hotline
pyrimethamine (Daraprim)	Burroughs Wellcome 1-800-722-9294	Financial assistance program
sargramostim (Prokine, GM-CSF)	Hoechst-Roussel 1-800-PROKINE	Financial assistance; indigent and uninsured program
trimethoprim-sulfa-methoxazole (Bactrim)	Burroughs 1-800-722-9294	Financial Wellcome assistance program
zalcitabine (Hivid, ddC)	Hoffman-LaRoche 1-800-285-4484	Financial assistance
zidovudine (Retrovir)	Burroughs Wellcome 1-800-722-9294	Financial assistance program

OTHER RESOURCES

AIDS Clinical Trials Information   Tel: 1-800-TRIALS-A
    Service
National Institutes of Health
Building 31, Room 7A32
Bethesda, Maryland 20850

American Foundation for AIDS   Tel: 1-212-682-7440
    Research
AM Far
733 3rd Avenue
1-800-722-9294

New York, NY 10017

Centers for Disease Control   Tel: 1-800-342-2437
    (CDC)
National AIDS Hotline

National AIDS Information   Tel: 1-800-458-5231
    Clearinghouse
P. O. Box 6003
Rockville, Maryland 20849-6003

National Information Center for   Tel: 1-800-336-4797
    Orphan Drugs and Rare
    Diseases

APPENDIX III

Quick Reference

I. CALCULATION OF ABSOLUTE NEUTROPHIL COUNT (ANC)

1. Total white blood count (WBC) multiplied by (sum of the neutrophils + bands divided by 100)

2. Lab results: WBC = $4000/mm^3$ (normal: 5000–$10,000/mm^3$)

neutrophils = 40	50–70%
bands = 2	
monocytes = 6	2–6%
eosinophils = 1	0.5–1%
lymphocytes = 50	20–40%

Total WBC (4000) X% (neut = 40 + bands = 2)
4000 X (40 + 2)/100
4000 X 0.42 = $1680/mm^3$

Normal ANC > $2000/mm^3$

3. Relative risk for infection related to ANC:

no significant risk	> 1500–$2000/mm^3$
minimal risk	1000–$1500/mm^3$
moderate risk	500–$1000/mm^3$
severe risk	< $500/mm^3$

Memory Bank for HIV Medications

II. CALCULATION OF URINE CREATININE CLEARANCE

Males estimated creatinine clearance $= \dfrac{(140 - \text{age}) \, (\text{weight in kg})}{72 \times \text{serum creatinine} \, (\text{mg/100 mL})}$

Females $= 0.85 \times$ estimated creatinine clearance of male

Source: Cockcroft DW, Gault MH (1976) Prediction of creatinine clearance from serum creatinine *Nephron* 16:31–41

III. BODY SURFACE AREA NOMOGRAM

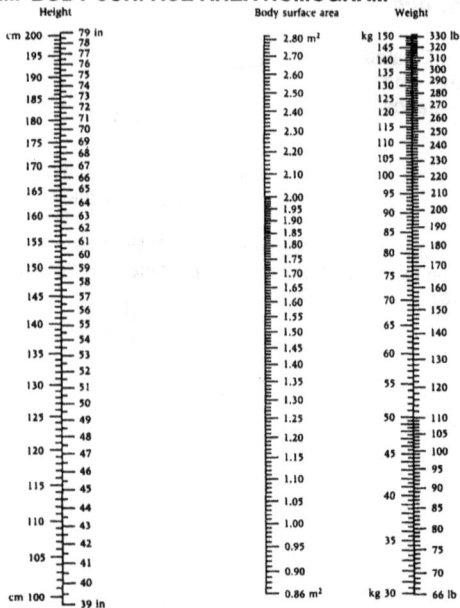

Height	Body surface area	Weight

To determine the BODY SURFACE AREA (BSA), find the height (in centimeters or inches) on the left hand column, then locate the weight (in kilograms or pounds) on the right column. Using a straight edge, connect the two columns at the identified points. The BSA is the point on the center column where the straight edge intersects. For example, a woman is 5 feet 5 inches tall (65 inches) and weighs 118 lbs. Her BSA is 1.4 m^2

Memory Bank for HIV Medications

APPENDIX IV

1993 Redbook
Average Wholesale Prices for
Drugs Commonly Used in the
Management of the Patient
with HIV Infection

Acetaminophen: 5 gr, 100 tabs $2.84
Acyclovir: 200 mg, 100 caps $88.49
Alprazolam: O.25 mg, 100 tabs $52.1 0
Amikacin: 500 mg/2mL vial $68.54
Amoxicillin/clavulanate: 250 mg, 30 tabs $51 .90
Amphotericin B: 50 mg vial, $37.06
Ampicillin: 500 mg vial, $3.20; 500 mg, 100 caps
   $7.37
Aspirin: 325 mg, 100 tabs $1 .09
Atovaquone: 250 mg, 200 tabs $511.20
Azithromycin: 250-mg, 30 tabs $205.26
Bleomycin: 15 unit vial, $256.19
Buspirone: 5 mg, 100 tabs $53.45
Butoconazole: 28 gm ointment, 1 tube $17.62
Capreomycin sulfate: 1 gm, $20.86
Cefamandole: 1 gm vial, $9.72
Cefixime: 200 mg, 100 tabs $240.63
Cefoxitin: 1 gm vial, $7.42
Ceftriaxone: 1 gm vial; 31.39
Cefuroxime axetil: 250 mg, 20 tabs $60.31
Chloral hydrate: 500 mg suppository, 100 supps
   $120.75
Chlorhexadine gluconate: 1 pint, $14.04

Source: Redbook (1993) Montvale, NJ: Medical
Economics Data Inc.

Clarithromycin: 250 mg, 60 tabs $160.36
Ciprofloxacin: 500 mg, 100 caps $292.25
Clindamycin hydrochloride: 150 mg caps, 100 $69.00
Clofazimine: 100 mg, 70 tabs $21.24
Clotrimazole: 10 mg, 70 loz $48.63
Codeine: 30 mg, 100 tabs $27.25
Cyclophosphamide: 1 gm vial, $49.11
Cycloserine: 250 mg, 40 tab $131.21
Cytosine arabinoside: 100 mg vial, $6.72
Dapsone: 100 mg, 100 tabs $18.00
Dexamethasone: 20 mg vial, $28.83
Didanosine: 100 mg, 60 tabs $86.42
Diphenhydramine: 50 mg, 100 caps $26.78
Diphenoxylate hydrochloride with atropine: 2.5 mg–
     0.025 mg, 100 tabs $40.71
Doxorubicn: 2Omg vial, $96.63
Doxycycline: 100 mg, 50 caps $157.05
Econazole nitrate: 15 gm tube of ointment, $10.62
Ethambutol hydrochloride: 100 mg, 100 tabs $38.62*
Ethionamide: 250 mg, 100 tab $146.95*
Epoetin: 3000 units/mL vial, $36.00 per vial
Erythrornycin: 250 mg, 100 tabs $31.00
Etoposide: 100 mg vial, $131.29
Filgastrim: 300 mcg/mL vial, $135.10 per vial
Fluoxetine hydrochloride: 20 mg, 100 tabs $201.47
Fluconazole: 100 mg, 30 caps $206.25;100 mg vial for
     IV, $81.30
Flucytosine: 250 mg, 100 tabs $100.30
Folinic acid: 25 mg, 25 tabs $600.00
Foscarnet: 250 mL (24 mg/mL), $73.28
Ganciclovir: 500 mg vial, $34.80
Griseofulvin: 25 mg, 100 tabs $3.45
Haloperidol: O.5 mg, 100 tabs $37.62
Hydrornorphone hydrochloride: 2 mg, 100 tabs
     $35.80

Ibuprofen: 400 mg, 100 tabs $3.75
Imipenern-cilastatin: 250 mg vial, $9.53
Interferon-alpha: 18 million unit vial, $162
Iodoquinol: 210 mg, 100 tabs $27.87
Isoniazid: 300 mg, 100 tabs $2.63*
Itraconazole: 100 mg, 30 tabs $147.60
Ketoconazole: 200 mg, 100 tabs $232.27
Kaolin-pectate: 1 pint, $3.90
Loperarnide: 2 mg, $50.57
Lorazepam: 1 mg, 100 tabs $2.48; 2 mg/mL IM/IV
   $11.51 per tubex
Megesterol acetate: 40 mg, 100 tabs $115.49
Meperidine: 50 mg tubex, $0.58 per tubex
Methadone: 5 mg, 100 tabs $6.04
Methotrexate: 250 mg vial, $26.88
Metronidazole: 250 mg, 50 tabs $62.91; 500 mg vial
   for IV, $15.53
Miconazole nitrate 2% cream: 1 oz, $5.20
Morphine sulfate: 10 mg/5 mL, 500 mL elixir, $20.00;
   10 mg supp, $1.00 each; MS Contin 30 mg, 50 tabs
   $69.74
Mupirocin 2% oint: 15 gm tube, $13.35
Naproxen: 250 mg, 100 tabs $71.53
Norfloxacin: 400 mg, 100 tabs $234.21
Nortriptyline: 25 mg, 100 tabs $69.79
Nystatin: 30 gm cream, $2.22; oral suspension,
   100,000u/mL, 60 mL $3.29; 100,000 unit tab, 15 tabs
   $2.78
Octreotide acetate: 50 mcg/mL, 1 mL vial $4.04
Ofloxacin: 200 mg, 50 caps $134.05
Ondansetron: 20 mL vial, $207.50 per vial
Oxycodone: Percocet® 100 tabs $63.56; Percodan)®
   100 tabs $65.63
Para-aminosalicylic acid: 100 mg, 100 tabs $4.50
Paromomycin sulfate: 250 mg, 16 tabs $27.61

Penicillin G Potassium: 250,000 unit tabs, 100 tabs $3.53; 1,000,000 units/vial for IV, 1 vial $1.27
Pentamidine, aerosolized: 300 mg vial, $85.00 per vial
Pentamidine, parenteral: 300 mg vial, $85.00 per vial
Pentoxifylline: 400 mg, 100 tabs $48.00
Permethrin 1% cream rinse: $8.18
Perphenazine: 4 mg, 100 tabs $37.73
Phenytoin: 100 mg, 100 caps $23.84
Podophyllum resin: 30 gm, $85.55
Podofilox 0.5%:   3.5 mL, $48.00
Prednisone: 50 mg, 100 tabs $15.28
Primaquine phosphate: 26.3 mg, 100 tabs $56.66
Probenecid: 500 mg, 100 tabs $12.50
Prochorperazine: 5 mg/2 mL, 2 mL vial $5.97; 25 mg supp, $2.50 ea; 10 mg spansule, 50 spansules $46.50
Pyrantel pamoate: 250 mg/5 mL, 60 mL vial $38.30
Pyrethrin blue gel: 1 oz, $1.84
Pyridoxine hydrochloride: 50 mg, 100 tabs $41.55*
Pyrimethamine: 25 mg, 100 tabs $34.75
Pyrazinamide: 500 mg, 100 tabs $92.97
Quinacrine hydrochloride: `   100 mg, 100 tabs $35.12
Retinoic acid 0.05%:   20 gm $24.66
Ritalin: 5 mg, 100 tabs $27.06
Rifabutin: 150 mg, 100 tabs $327.00
Rifampin: 300 mg, 100 tabs $204.06*
Sargramostrim: 250 mcg/vial, 1 vial $106.00
Spectinomycin dihydrochloride: 2 gm vial, $14.25
Spiramycin: investigational agent
Stavudine: investigational agent
Streptomycin sulfate: 25 gm powder, $17.25
Sulbactam:.investigational agent
Sulfadiazine: 500 mg, 100 tabs $9.60
Terconazole 0.4% cream: 45 gm $21.30

Thiabendazole: 500 mg, 36 tabs $32.95
Tioconazole 6.5% ointment: 4.6 gm, $23.06
Trazodone hydrochloride: 50 mg, 100 tabs $114.35
Trimethoprim: 100 mg, 100 tabs $19.13
Trimethoprim-sulfamethoxazole: Bactrim® DS, 100 tabs $113.30
Trimetrexate gluconate: investigational, free under treatment IND
Vancomycin hydrochloride: 1 gm vial, $1 5.60
Vinblastine sulfate: 10 mg vial, $35.24
Vincristine sulfate: 1 mg vial, $29.50
Zalcitabine: O.75O mg, 100 tabs $213.60
Zidovudine: 100 mg, 100 caps $144.23

*Free from most community Departments of Public Health

These are the average wholesale prices (AWP) as indicated for generic drug or trade name of drug. Hospital or retail pharmacies may double or triple this price when dispensing the drug to the patient. However, many pharmaceutical companies provide indigent programs, providing free or low cost drug to patients without insurance or economic means. In addition, some AIDSactivist groups have developed resource organizations that provide free medications to indigent patients.

Aerosolized pentamidine requires a nebulizer to administer the drug. Comparative 1993 prices for the three commonly used nebulizers are:

Respirgard II	$124/month
Aerotech II	62/month
Fisoneb	40/month

Nebulizer cost $400 to $500 to purchase

Appendix IV   **339**

BIBLIOGRAPHY

Aboulker JP, Swart AM (1993) Report of Concorde I
    Study of zidovudine in asymptomatic HIV-seropositive
    patients *Lancet* 341:889–890
Abramowicz M (1993) Itraconazole *The Medical Letter*
    35(888):7–9
Ames ED, Conjalka MS, Goldberg AF et al (1991)
    Hodgkin's disease and AIDS *Hematol Oncol Clin
    North Am* 5:343–356
Bartlett JG (1993) *The Johns Hopkins Hospital Guide to
    medical care of patients with HIV infection*, 3rd
    Edition. Baltimore, MD: Williams and Wilkins
Bartlett JG (1993) *Pocketbook of infectious disease
    therapy* Baltimore, MD: Williams and Wilkins
Bozzette SA, Sattler FR, Chiu J et al (1990) A controlled
    trial of early adjunctive treatment of corticosteroids for
    Pneumocystis carinii pneumonia in acquired
    immunodeficiency syndrome *NEJM* 323:1451–1457
Buckley RM, Braffman MN, Stern JJ (1990) Opportunistic
    Infections in the Acquired immunodeficiency
    syndrome *Seminars in Oncology* 17(3):335–349
Carr A, Tindall B, Brew BJ et al (1991) Low-dose
    trimethoprim-sulfamethoxazole prophylaxis for
    toxoplasmosis encephalitis in patients with AIDS *Ann
    Intern Med* 117:106–111
Centers for Disease Control (1990) Risk for cervical
    disease in HIV-infected women in New York City
    MMWR 39:846–849

Centers for Disease Control (1989) Recommendations of
the Immunization Practices Advisory Committee:
Pneumococcal polysaccharide vaccine *MMWR*
38:64–76

Centers for Disease Control (1991) Purified protein
derivative (PPD) tuberculin anergy and HIV infection:
guidelines for anergy testing and management of
anergic persons at risk for tuberculosis *MMWR*
40(RR-5):27–33

Centers for Disease Control (¡992) Prevention and
Control of influenza recommendations of the
Immunization Practice Advisory Committee *MMWR*
41(RR-9):1–17

Centers for Disease Control (1992) 1993 revised
classification system for HIV infection and expanded
surveillance case definition for AIDS among
adolescents and adults *MMWR* 41(RR-17)1–19

Centers for Disease Control (1992) Recommendations
for prophylaxis against Pneumocystis carinii
pneumonia for adults and adolescents infected with
HIV *MMWR* 41(RR-4):1–11

Chiu J, Nussbaum J, Bozzette S et al (1990) Treatment
of Disseminated Mycobacterium avium complex
infection in AIDS patients with amikacin, ethambutol,
rifampin, and ciprofloxacin *Ann Intern Med*
113(5):358–361

Cohen PT, Sande MA, Volberding PA (EDs) (1990) *The
AIDS knowledge base: a textbook on HIV disease*.
Waltham, MA: Medical Publishing Group

Cohn DL, Hosburgh CR (1993) Treatment and prophylaxis of disseminated Mycobacterium avium complex infection in AIDS *Opportunistic complications of HIV* 2(1):9–11

Cooley T (1993) *AIDS-related non-Hodgkin's lymphoma*, Ch 27, in H Libman and R Witzburg (Eds), *HIV Infection: A Clinical Manual.* Boston: Little Brown

Cooley T (1993) *Kaposi's Sarcoma,* Ch 26, In H Libman and R Witzburg (Eds),*HIV infection: A Clinical Manual,* Boston: Little, Brown

Cooley T, Kunches LM, Saunders C et al (1990) Treatment of AIDS and AIDS-related complex with 2',3'-dideoxyinosine given once daily. *Reviews of Infect Dis* 12(Suppl 5):S552–560

Ellerbrock TV, and Rogers MF (1990) Epidemiology of human immunodeficiency virus infection in women in the United States *Obstetrics and Gynecology of North America* 17:523–543

Erlich KS, Mills J, Chatis P et al (1989) Acyclovir-resistant herpes simplex virus infections in patients with AIDS *NEJM* 320(5):293–296

Fazely F (1991) Pentotoxifylline (Trentyl) decreases the replication of HIV-1 in human peripheral blood mononuclear cells and in cultured T-cells *Blood* 77:1653–1656

Gill PS, Rarick M, McCutchan JA et al (1991) Systemic treatment of AIDS-related Kaposi's Sarcoma: results of a randomized trial *Am J Med* 90:427–433

Griffiths PD (1990) Virus infections in patients with AIDS *Transactions of the Royal Soc of Trop Med and Hygiene 84(Suppl 1):7–8 Hygiene*

Groopman JE (1987) Neoplasms in the acquired immunodeficiency syndrome: the multidisciplinary approach to treatment *Seminars in Oncology* 14(2):1–6 (Suppl 3)

Groopman JE, Scadden DT (1989) Interferon therapy for Kaposi's sarcoma associated with the acquired immunodeficiency syndrome *Ann Inter Med* 110:335–337

Hadler SC (1988) Hepatitis B prevention and HIV infection *Annals of Int Med* 109:92–94

Hardy WD (1992) A controlled trial of trimethoprim-sulfamethoxazole or aerosolized pentamidine for secondary prophylaxis in patients with AIDS: AIDS clinical trials group protocol 021 *NEJM* 327:1842–1848

Hughes WT, Kennedy W, Dugdale M et al (1990) Prevention of Pneumocytis carinii pneumonitis in AIDS patients with weekly dapsone *Lancet* 336:1066

Jacob JL, Baird BF, Haller S, and Ostchega Y (1989) AIDS-Related Kaposi's sarcoma: concepts of care *Seminars in Oncology Nursing* 5(4):263–275

Jewett JF, Hecht FM (1993) Preventative health care for adults with HIV infection *JAMA* 269(9):1144–1153

Kaplan LD, Abrams DI, Feigal E et al (1989) AIDS associated non-Hodgkin's lymphoma in San Francisco *JAMA* 261:719–724

Kaplan LD, Kahn JO, Crowe S et al (1991) Clinical and virologic effects of rGM-CSF in patients receiving chemotherapy for HIV-associated non-Hodgkin's lymphoma *J Clin Oncol 9:929–940*

Koda-Kimball MA, Young LY (eds) (1992) *Applied therapeutics: the clinical use of drugs* Vancouver: Applied therapeutics *AIDS* 2:71–80

Koonin LM, Ellerbrock TV, Atrash HK et al (1989) Pregnancy associated deaths due to AIDS in the United States *JAMA* 261:1306–1309

Krown SE (1988) AIDS-associated Kaposi's sarcoma: pathogenesis, clinical course and treatment *AIDS* 2:71–80

Krown SE, Metroka C, Werntz JC (1989) AIDS Clinical Trials Group Oncology Committee, Kaposi's sarcoma in the acquired immune deficiency syndrome: a proposal for uniform evaluation, response and staging criteria *J Clin Oncol* 7:1201–1207

Lake-Bakaar G, Tom W, Lake-Bakaar D et al (1988) Gastropathy and ketoconazole malabsorption in the acquired immune deficiency syndrome *Ann Intern Med* 109:471–473

Lavelle J, Falloon J, Morgan A et al (1991) Weekly dapsone and dapsone/pyrimethamine for pneumocystic carinii pneumonia prophylaxis *Abstract WB 2207*, in *Program and abstract of the Vii International Conference on AIDS*, Florence, 1991

Lee BLL, Safrin S (1992) Interactions and toxicities of drugs used in patients with AIDS *Clin Infect Dis* 14:773–779

Levine AM (1987) Non-Hodgkin's Lymphomas and other malignancies in the acquired immune deficiency syndrome *Seminars in Oncology* 14(2):34–39 (Suppl 3)

Levine AM (1989) Low-dose chemotherapy with CNS prophylaxis and zidovudine maintenance for AIDS-related lymphoma *Blood* 74(Suppl 1):239

Levine SL, Masur H, Gill VJ et al (1991) The effects of aerosolized pentamidine prophylaxis on the diagnosis of Pneumocystis carinii pneumonia by induced sputum exam in patients infected with HIV *Ann Rev Respir Dis* 144:760–764

Lucey DR, Hensley RE, Ward WW et al (1991) CD4+ monocyte counts in persons with HIV-1 infection: an early increase is followed by a progressive decline *J Acquired Immunodef Syndrome* 4(1):24–31

MacDonell KB and Glassroth J (1989) Mycobacterium avium complex and other nontuberculous mycobacteria in patients with HIV infection *Seminars in Respir Infections* 4(2):123–132

McCabe RE (1990) Current diagnosis and management of toxoplasmosis in cancer patients *Oncology* 4(10):81–94

McEnvoy GK, Litvak K, Welsh OH et al (EDs)(1993) *AHFS drug information, 1993* Bethesda, MD: Am Soc of Hosp Pharm

Montgomery AB, Debs RJ, Luce JM et al (1988) Selective delivery of pentamidine to the lung by aerosolization *Am Rev Respir Dis*137:477–478

Moss AR, Bacchetti P (1989) Natural history of HIV infection *J Acquired Immunodef Syndrome* 3(2):55–61

Nursing 93 drug handbook (1992) Springhouse, PA: Springhous Corp

Physician's drug reference (1993) Montvale, NJ: Medical Economics Corp

Red Book (1993) Montvale, NJ: Medical Economics Data Inc

Sande MA,Volberding PA (Eds) (1992) *Medical management of AIDS,* 3rd Edition.Philadelphia, PA: WB Saunders

Sanford JP, Sande MA, Gilbert DN, Gerberding JL (1992) *The Sanford guide to HIV/AIDS therapy* Dallas, Tx: Antimicrobial Therapy Inc

Santangelo J, Schnack J (1991) Primary care intervention and management for adults with early HIV infection *Nurse Practitioner* 16(6):9–15

Sewester CS, Olin BR, Hebel SK et al (Eds) (1991) *Drug facts and comparisons 1991* St Louis, MO: JB Lippincott

Shepherd FA, Evans WK, Garvey B et al (1988) Combination chemotherapy and alpha-interferon in the treatment of kaposi's sarcoma associated with acquired immune deficiency syndrome *CMAJ* 139:635–639

Skowron G, Merigan TC (1990) Alternating and intermittent regimens of zidovudine and dideoxycytidine in the treatment of patients with AIDS and ARC *Am J Med* 88 (Suppl 5B):205–235

Sugar AM, Saunders C (1988) Oral fluconazole as suppression therapy of disseminated cryptococcosis in AIDS *Ann Int Med* 85:481–489

Tinkle MB, Amaya MA, Tamayo OW (1992) HIV disease and pregnancy Part I *JOGNN* 21(2):86–93

Tsivitis MC (1993) Resurgent tuberculosis *Cancer Practice* 1(3):233–240

Unger PD, Stranchen JA (1986) Hodgkin's disease in AIDS-related complex patients *Cancer* 58:821–825

U.S. Public Health Service Task Force on antipneumocystis prophylaxis in patients with HIV infection (1993) Recommendations for prophylaxis *J Acq Immunodef Synd* 6(1):46–55

U.S. Public Health Service(1990) State of the Art

Conference on azidothymidine therapy for early HIV infection *Am J Med* 89:335–344

Valentine FT (1990) Pathogenesis of the immunological deficiencies caused by infection with the Human Immunodeficiecy virus *Seminars in Oncology* 17(3)321–334

Vogel J (1988) The HIV tat gene induces dermal lesions resembling kaposi's sarcoma in transgenic mice *Nature* 335:606–611

Volberding P, Lagakos F, Fischl M et al (1990) Zidovudine in asymptomatic HIV infection: a controlled trial in persons with <500 CD4+ cells/mm3 *NEJM* 322(14): 941–948

Walsh C, Wernz JC, Levine A et al (1993) Phase 1 Trial of m-BACOD and granulocyte-acrophage colony stimulating factor in HIV-associated non-Hodgkin's Lymphoma *J Acquired Immunodef Syndrome* 6(3):265–271

Wilkes GM (1992) Polypharmacy: dangers of multiple-drug therapy in patients with HIV infection *Home Healthcare Nurse* 10(5):30–47

Wilkes GM, Igwersen K, Burke MB (1993) *Oncology nursing drug reference* Boston: Jones and Bartlett

Wormser GP, Horowitz HW, Duncanson FP et al (1991) Low dose intermittent trimethoprim-sulfamethoxazole for prevention of pneumocystis carinii pneumonia in patients with HIV infection *Arch Intern Med* 151:688–692

Index

Diphenhydramine hydrochloride, 110
Diphenoxylate hydrochloride and atropine, 112
Diquinol, 159
Dolophine, 183
Doryx, 116
Doxorubicin, 31, 114
Doxy-Caps, 116
Doxycycline hydrochloride, 116
Duramorph, 196

E

E-mycin, 126
Econazole nitrate1% cream, 118
Ecotrin, 49
Elimite 5% cream, 235
Epoetin alfa, 124
Erythromycin base, 126
Ethambutol, 19
Ethambutol hydrochloride, 120
Ethionamide, 122
Etoposide, 128

F

Femstat, 61
Filgrastim, 130
Flagyl, 191

Floxin, 213
Fluconazole, 132
Flucytosine, 134
Fluoxetine hydrochloride, 137
Folex, 186
Folinic acid, 172
Foscarnet, 139
Foscavir, 139
Fulvicin, 145
Fungal infections, 23
Fungizone, 44

G

G-CSF, 130
Ganciclovir, 142
GM-CSF, 29, 273
Grifulvin, 145
Gris-PEG, 145
Grisactin, 145
Griseofulvin, 145
Gyne-Lotrimin vaginal cream, 89

H

Hairy leukoplakia, 23
Haldol, 148
Haloperidol, 148
Herpes simplex virus (HSV), 21
Hexa-betalin, 260

RID lice killing shampoo,
    259
Rifabutin, 267
Rifadin, 270
Rifampin, 18, 270
Ritalin SR, 189
Robimycin, 126
Robitabs, 126
Rodex, 260
Roferon-A, 156
Rovamycine, 279
Roxanol, 196
Roxicodone, 218
Rufen, 152

S

Sandostatin, 211
Sargramostim, 273
Septra, 297
Septra DS, 297
Seromycin pulvules, 96
Shingles, 22
Spectazole (with benzoic
    acid), 118
Spectinomycin
    dihydrochloride, 276
Spiramycin, 279
Sporanox, 165
Stavudine, 280
Streptomycin sulfate, 281
Sulbactam, 284
Sulfadiazine, 27, 285

Sulfamethoprim, 297
Suprax, 67

T

Terconazole, 288
Thiabendazole, 290
Tioconazole 6.5%, 292
TMP-SMX, 25, 297
Toxoplasma gondii, 26
Toxoplasmosis, 25
Trazodone hydrochloride,
    293
Trecator-SC, 122
Trentyl, 233
Trilafon, 237
Trimethoprim, 26
Trimethoprim and
    sulfamethoxazole,
    297
Trimethoprim sulfate, 295
Trimetrexate gluconate,
    301
Trimpex, 295
Trobicin , 276
Tubasal, 221
Tuberculosis, 17
Tubizid, 162
Tylenol, 33

V

Vaginal creams, 288

www.ingramcontent.com/pod-product-compliance
Lightning Source LLC
Chambersburg PA
CBHW060759220326
41598CB00022B/2485